Psychological Treatment of Panic

TREATMENT MANUALS FOR PRACTITIONERS
David H. Barlow, *Editor*

PSYCHOLOGICAL TREATMENT OF PANIC
David H. Barlow and Jerome A. Cerny

Forthcoming
SELF-MANAGEMENT PROGRAM FOR TROUBLED ADOLESCENTS
Thomas A. Brigham

Psychological Treatment of Panic

DAVID H. BARLOW
State University of New York at Albany

JEROME A. CERNY
Indiana State University

THE GUILFORD PRESS
New York London

© 1988 The Guilford Press
A Division of Guilford Publications, Inc.
72 Spring Street, New York, NY 10012

Printed in the United States of America

Last digit is print number: 9 8 7 6 5 4

Library of Congress Cataloging-in-Publication Data
Barlow, David H.
   Psychological treatment of panic.
   (Treatment manuals for practitioners)
   Bibliography: p.
   Includes index.
   1. Panic disorders—Treatment.   2. Behavior therapy.
I. Cerny, Jerome A.   II. Title.   III. Series
RC535.B28   1988   616.85′223   87-19682
ISBN 0-89862-203-4 (cloth)
ISBN 0-89862-507-6 (paper)

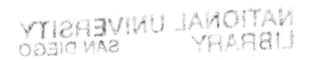

For Bob Lanigan, a friend for over 30 years.

And to Burke and Derek Cerny,
and to all our students, staff, and clients,
who helped shape our ideas and practice.

Preface

The purpose of this book is to describe a step-by-step treatment protocol for panic disorder. Two developments made this book both possible and necessary. First, the development of successful problem-oriented treatments for specific psychological disorders has created an enormous need for dissemination of these treatment programs to mental health professionals. It is not enough to simply review the literature and note that recent research indicates that a new treatment is successful with a specific disorder. Professionals want to know how to do it. Answering this question necessarily involves illustrating treatment programs in minute detail. Many important steps that are taken for granted by the developers of these programs only become obvious when treatment programs are illustrated in a very systematic fashion. This book attempts to fulfill that purpose for panic disorder.

Second, one of the newest developments within the psychosocial treatment of emotional and behavioral disorders is the treatment of panic. In the context of wide publicity over drug treatments for these problems, few practitioners are even aware that successful psychosocial treatments exist. For that reason, it seems important not only to review evidence for the effectiveness of these approaches, but also to present in a detailed fashion the nuts and bolts of this treatment. In this way, mental health practitioners preferring nondrug approaches will have these tools at their disposal. Similarly, clients burdened by debilitating panic attacks will have an increased number of treatment options. The fact that initial evidence suggests that these treatments are extremely successful for panic makes dissemination of this information all the more important. Thus, the purpose of this book is to present our newly developed cognitive-behavioral treatment of panic with enough detail to allow trained clinicians generally familiar with this approach to incorporate this program immediately into their therapeutic armamentarium.

In accomplishing this goal we owe a considerable debt of gratitude to Leigh Petronis, Wendy Rapee, and Jane Richardson, who spent long hours typing and editing the manuscript under what seemed to be impossible deadlines. Our thanks also to Jeremy C. Barlow for some observations on Greek mythology, and to Rhonda Salge, David Williams, and Cindy Lopatka for compiling a useful index. Finally, we certainly want to acknowledge that treatments such as the one presented in this book do not develop in a vacuum. The National Institute of Mental Health supported the clinical research that led directly to the development of this treatment. Countless discussions and interchanges with our colleagues from around the world working in the anxiety disorders influenced our research directions. Doctoral students in clinical psychology participating in our clinical research projects made numerous valuable suggestions as this treatment was in construction. While we take full responsibility for any flaws in this first-generation psychosocial treatment of panic, we acknowledge, with gratitude, all of the contributions to what appears to be a successful new treatment.

Contents

Psychological Treatment of Panic

1

The Nature and Consequences of Panic

The roots of the experience of panic are deeply embedded in our cultural myths. Pan, the Greek god of nature, resided in the countryside presiding over rivers, woods, streams, and the various grazing animals. But Pan did not fit the popular image of a god. He was very short with legs resembling those of a goat. And he was very ugly. Pan also habitually napped in a small cave or thicket near the road. If a luckless ancient Greek traveler disturbed Pan's nap, Pan would let out a blood-curdling scream that was said to make one's hair stand on end. Pan's scream was so intense that many a terrified traveler died. This sudden overwhelming terror or fright came to be known as *panic*, and on occasion, Pan would use his unique talent to vanquish his foes. Even the gods themselves were subject to his terror and at his mercy.

While Pan has faded deep into myth, his power is experienced daily by millions. In fact, panic may be so common, so widespread, and so much a part of our experience that we have managed to overlook its importance. In lay terms, "panicking" is a part of our life; usually occurring before some deadline that seems impossible to make, or when suddenly faced with danger. But understanding the phenomenon of panic may be essential if we are to solve the many puzzles surrounding anxiety disorders. In addition, we now know that a full understanding of other major psychological disorders (such as depression, somatoform disorders, and stress disorders) may be difficult without first understanding panic. And yet we know very little about the phenomenon of panic.

The Presentation of Panic

Much of our recent increased attention to the concept of panic is due to the description of panic in the third edition of the *Diagnostic and Statistical Manual of Mental Disorders* (DSM-III) (American Psychiatric Association, 1980), where it was defined as "the sudden onset of intense apprehension, fear or terror, often associated with feelings of impending doom" (pp. 230). "Sudden onset" has come to mean 10 minutes during which panic will reach a peak, and this temporal criterion is included in the revision of DSM-III (DSM-III-R) (American Psychiatric Association, 1987).

Serendipitous physiological recording of unexpected panic has been reported at the Center for Stress and Anxiety Disorders, State University of New York at Albany (Cohen, Barlow, & Blanchard, 1985). We recorded the responses of two subjects who panicked during the relaxation phase of a standard physiological assessment. The physiological profiles were very similar, as evident from Figures 1-1 and 1-2. Initial decreases in heart rate and electromyographic (EMG) measures indicated that the subjects were beginning to relax. These decreases were followed by abrupt increases, reaching a level of tachycardia within 1 minute for one subject and within 2 minutes for the other subject. EMG measures also increased during the panic episodes for both patients. Hand surface temperature change was consistent across both subjects, showing an abrupt increase during panic, a pattern that differs from the usual finding of a decrease in peripheral temperature during stress. Findings such as this support the "sudden onset" criterion for panic.

A second important part of the definition is the list of symptoms that constitute a panic attack. Most of these symptoms are physical or somatic expressions of panic such as palpitations or dizziness. DSM-III listed 12 symptoms and specified that at least 4 must be present to label the event a true, or full-blown, panic attack. In DSM-III-R, 14 symptoms are listed (see Table 1-1). This is accomplished by adding one somatic symptom (nausea or abdominal distress) and by breaking down the DSM-III symptom 12—fear of dying, going crazy, or doing something uncontrolled during an attack—into two symptoms: (1) fear of dying, and (2) fear of going crazy or doing something uncontrolled. This allows a bit more precision in identifying the characteristic physical symptoms as well as the cognitive expression of dread (going crazy or dying) that an individual may present during a panic attack. Once again, this individual must report having a panic characterized by "the sudden onset of intense apprehension," and so on, *and* report at least four of these symptoms.

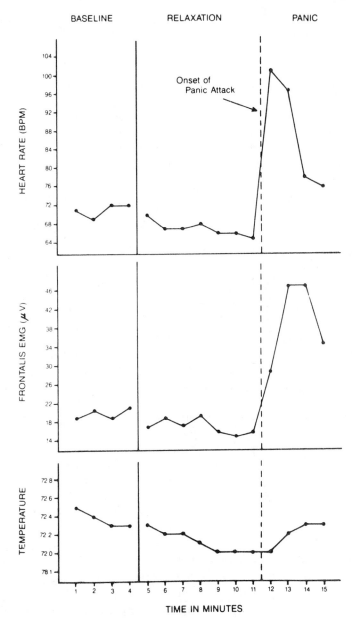

FIGURE 1-1. Heart rate (beats per minute; BPM), average integrated electromyogram (EMG), and hand-surface temperature for Subject 1. Reprinted with permission from: Cohen, A. S., Barlow, D. H., & Blanchard, E. B. The psychophysiology of relaxation-associated panic attacks. *Journal of Abnormal Psychology*, 1985, *94*, 96–101. Copyright 1985 by the American Psychological Association.

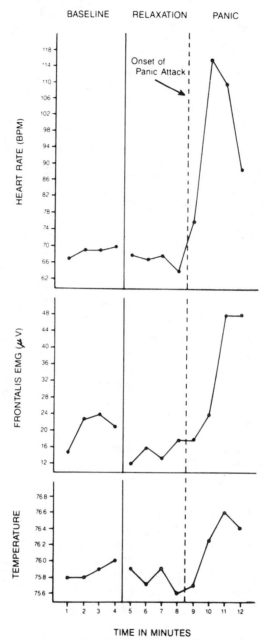

TIME IN MINUTES

FIGURE 1-2. Heart rate, average integrated electromyogram (EMG), and hand-surface temperature for Subject 2. Reprinted with permission from: Cohen, A. S., Barlow, D. H., & Blanchard, E. B. The psychophysiology of relaxation-associated panic attacks. *Journal of Abnormal Psychology*, 1985, *94*, 96–101. Copyright 1985 by the American Psychological Association.

TABLE 1-1. List of DSM-III-R Panic Symptoms

1. Shortness of breath (dyspnea) or smothering sensations
2. Choking
3. Palpitations or accelerated heart rate (tachycardia)
4. Chest pain or discomfort
5. Sweating
6. Faintness
7. Dizziness, lightheadedness, or unsteady feelings
8. Nausea or abdominal distress
9. Depersonalization or derealization
10. Numbness or tingling sensations (paresthesias)
11. Flushes (hot flashes) or chills
12. Trembling or shaking
13. Fear of dying
14. Fear of going crazy or doing something uncontrolled

Note. Reprinted with permission from the *Diagnositc and Statistical Manual of Mental Disorders, Third Edition, Revised.* Copyright 1987 American Psychiatric Association.

These symptoms were identified largely through the clinical experience of investigators working with anxiety disorders. Clinical experience also tells us both that different individuals may experience different combinations of the symptoms and that even the same person may report a slightly different mix of symptoms from one panic attack to another. Most clients who are experiencing panic attacks usually report far more than the minimum number of four symptoms specified in DSM-III or DSM-III-R. Recently, we asked a large group of panic disorder clients (most with substantial agoraphobic avoidance) which symptoms each of them experienced during their typical or most recent panic attack (Barlow *et al.,* 1985). Table 1-2 lists both the number and the percentage of agoraphobics with panic ($N = 41$) who cited each of the 12 DSM-III symptoms.

Almost all of these clients reported palpitations and dizziness. In addition, 90% or more also reported fear of going crazy or losing control, as well as the symptoms of sweating and shortness of breath (dyspnea). Fear of going crazy or losing control represents the cognitive consequence of being afraid of panic. Because these descriptions were taken mostly from their typical panics, the specific number of symptoms associated with any one discrete panic experience may be somewhat fewer.

Limited Symptom Attacks

Clinicians have identified what seems to be another variety of panic attack that meets all the aforementioned criteria for panic with one

TABLE 1-2. Number and Percentage of 41 Agoraphobics with Panic Reporting Each of the DSM-III Panic Symptoms

Symptom	Agoraphobia with panic (N = 41)	
	Number	%
Dyspnea	37	90%
Palpitations	40	98%
Chest pain	31	76%
Choking	30	73%
Dizziness	39	95%
Feeling of unreality	28	68%
Paresthesias	26	63%
Hot or cold flashes	35	85%
Sweating	35	93%
Faintness	31	76%
Trembling	36	88%
Fear of going crazy or losing control	37	90%

Note. Adapted from Barlow et al. (1985).

exception: Fewer than four symptoms were reported. In DSM-III-R these experiences are called limited symptom attacks. In other places, such as the large Upjohn-sponsored cross-national study on the effectiveness of alprazolam for panic, they are referred to as minor attacks. We now have evidence that these minor attacks are aptly named because, on the whole, they are rated by clients as less intense than major attacks (Taylor et al., 1986).

This diminished intensity is not always the case, however. For example, we recently saw a woman who reported that her initial panic episode consisted of two specific symptoms: diarrhea and excessive perspiration. Following that first episode, a typical agoraphobic pattern emerged in which she would avoid going out as much as possible. Her greatest fear was that the diarrhea and sweating would suddenly recur (which would occasionally happen). Thus, when she did go out, she would always check for the availability of bathrooms, and would only begin to feel more comfortable when she had easy access to a bathroom. She also paid particular attention to the wearing of antiperspirants and so on. This woman soon learned the location of every bathroom along her frequented routes in the small city in which she lived.

Functionally, this experience seems to serve the same purpose as a panic attack. That is, it has the same consequences in terms of development of anxiety and avoidance. However, in our clinical experience, this type of attack is relatively rare in the absence of full-blown panic attacks. For example, in the aforementioned series of 41 agoraphobics, only 1 person reported these limited attacks without ever having experienced a full-blown attack.

On the other hand, clients who experience a full-blown panic may have a number of these minor attacks. For example, while self-monitoring panics for 6 days, 24 hours a day, Taylor *et al.* (1986) noted that in a group of 12 clients with panic disorder, 8 out of 33 panic attacks would be classified as minor or limited symptom attacks. However, criteria from the Upjohn cross-national collaborative study were used in this investigation. Specifically, only three rather than four symptoms were required to qualify an attack as major, which left only reports of one or two symptoms eligible for the minor category. If DSM-III criteria were used, and attacks with three symptoms were also counted as limited attacks, the percentage of limited attacks might be higher. Nevertheless, on a scale of 0 to 7, these limited attacks were rated by patients at an average intensity of 2.5 compared to 3.9 for full-blown attacks and were associated with average heart rate increases of 17.3 beats per minute (BPM) as compared to a 49.2 BPM increase for major attacks.

In summary, panic attacks are described as sudden bursts of emotion consisting of a large number of somatic symptoms and feelings of dying and/or losing control. The symptoms are relatively consistent on the average across people experiencing panic, but individual panic attacks may present with a different mix of symptoms, fewer symptoms, or variations in intensity of symptoms.

The Uniqueness of Panic

Is panic unique? The uniqueness of panic is an area of intense study and speculation. Justification for differentiating panic from intense generalized anxiety is supported by four methods of analysis, each of which falls short in some respects.

Pharmacological Dissection

The first of these methods involves the observation of differential response to drug treatment in a method that has come to be known as "pharmacological dissection." This method was first reported by Donald Klein and his colleagues (Klein & Fink, 1962; Klein, 1964). In early work designed to test the effectiveness of a drug called imipramine, Klein observed that this drug semed to reduce or eliminate panic attacks but had little effect on chronic levels of anticipatory anxiety. On that basis, he assumed that panic attacks were not simply severe states of general anxiety. Klein thus "dissected" panic attacks from generalized, chronic or anticipatory anxiety as a qualitatively different state (Klein & Fink, 1962; Klein, 1964). Unfortunately, his reasoning was based on the logical fallacy of inferring pretreatment differences from treatment effects. Also, it now seems that any number of pharmacological agents may be effective for panic (Liebowitz, 1985). However, Klein's work did suggest directions for future research.

Psychological Dissection

The second method may be termed "psychological dissection." Waddell, Barlow, and O'Brien (1984) studied the differential treatment effects of a combined treatment program on chronic background anxiety and panic attacks. In their multiple-baseline across-subjects design, three subjects were treated sequentially with (1) relaxation training and (2) cognitive restructuring. The clients self-monitored both number and duration of episodes of intense anxiety and panic, rated as 4 or higher on a scale of 0 to 8. In addition, they recorded their subjectively experienced level of general anxiety four times each day. All three clients demonstrated marked decreases in the number of episodes of intense anxiety and panic, an improvement that was maintained at a 3-month follow-up. However, two clients exhibited a clear increase in background anxiety at the same time that episodes of intense anxiety and panic were reduced. The third client demonstrated synchronous reductions in background anxiety and episodes of panic.

It is tempting to conclude from these results that there are two different types of anxiety that respond differentially to the same treatment procedures. In so doing, however, one commits the same logical error for which Klein was criticized. In addition, the data are limited to three clients in whom a consistent pattern of differentiation between panic and chronic anxiety was not present. Further, these data do not exclude the possibilities both that panic and chronic anxiety differ quantitatively but not qualitatively and that the impact of psychological and pharmocological treatment is only noticeable in the case of intense levels of anxiety. Moreover, a set of data collected recently from a group of 16 clients with panic disorder (who underwent a comprehensive treatment at the Phobia and Anxiety Disorders Clinic) indicated that both the number of panic attacks and the general anxiety ratings decreased from pre- to postassessment: Mean number of panic attacks per week decreased from 1.31 to 0.10, and mean anxiety ratings decreased from 2.31 to 1.37 (Klosko & Barlow, 1987). However, group averages mask individual patterns of response, and it is likely that some clients within that group did not experience parallel changes in panic and generalized anxiety.

Neurobiology and Genetics

The third method reaches broadly and deeply into the areas of behavioral genetics and neurobiology to search for differential biological and genetic underpinnings to panic and generalized anxiety. (See Barlow, 1988, for a detailed discussion of this issue.) Suffice it to say here that exciting neurobiological research concerning neurotransmitters and their various receptor systems is continuing as investigators attempt to isolate the biological basis of panic. Nevertheless, there has not yet been a discovery of a clear biological marker for panic, as every speculative hypothesis on differential neurobiological processes has failed rigorous empirical tests (Barlow, 1988; Charney, Woods, Goodman, & Heninger, 1985; Margraf, Ehlers, & Roth, 1986).

A seemingly more promising line of investigation has examined the genetic basis of panic. After early retrospective studies suggesting different family backgrounds in panic disorder versus generalized anxiety disorder (e.g., Raskin, Peeke, Dickman, & Pinkster, 1982), a number of studies attempted to investigate more systematically differential family aggregation of panic (e.g., Crowe, Noyes, Pauls, & Slymen, 1983; Harris, Noyes, Crowe, & Chaudry, 1983; Moran & Andrews, 1985). Other studies have examined more directly the genetic basis of panic using twin-study methodology (Torgerson, 1983a). All of these studies found that panic aggregated in families or in monozygotic twins whereas generalized anxiety did not.

In fact, we have known for a long time that clinical anxiety seems to run in families and is probably at least partially inherited (Brown, 1942; Carey & Gottesman, 1981; Cohen, Badal, Kilpatrick, Reed, & White, 1951; Slater & Shields, 1969). We are also quite sure that the personality trait that has been termed "neuroticism" or "emotionality" runs in families and probably has a genetic component (Broadhurst, 1975; Gray, 1982). What is new about the more recent studies, then, is the suggestion that panic is hereditable, whereas generalized anxiety is not. This information is directly at odds with all early studies unless the early studies were only assessing people with panic who were classified under broader headings in use at the time (such as "anxiety neurosis"), something that is impossible to ascertain at this time. Even this, however, would not account for the hereditability of an "anxious" personality.

Because findings for a specific genetic component to panic, as opposed to generalized anxiety are very much at odds with a broader view of the hereditability of anxiety, often referred to as nervousness or emotionality, it is possible that these results are artifactual. In addition to major methodological problems with existing work (Carey & Gottesman, 1981; Carey, 1985), a close examination of this literature reveals one very clear artifact that might make this finding spurious.

First, studies supporting the hypothetical differential genetic contribution to panic and generalized anxiety utilized DSM-III diagnostic criteria. But there is a diagnostic convention in DSM-III (not present in DSM-III-R) that generalized anxiety disorder is a residual category to be diagnosed only in the absence of any other anxiety-based symptoms such as panic, phobic avoidance, or obsessive thoughts. In fact, data indicate that almost all individuals with panic disorder also present with marked "generalized anxiety" (Barlow, Blanchard, Vermilyea, Vermilyea, & Di Nardo, 1986). Therefore, the only subjects included in the category "generalized anxiety disorder" in the Crowe et al. (1983) study, for example, were those not panicking at all. It is almost certain that these were less severe cases.

In Torgerson's (1983a) twin study, commonly regarded as the strongest supporting evidence for differential hereditability of a panic, a genetic contribution to neurotic disorders was found only among those probands who were inpatients and not those who were outpatients. Once again this may be reflecting the influence of severity on hereditability rather than differential anxiety symptoms. Cloninger, Martin, Clayton, and Guze (1981), in sketching out the natural history of panic disorder, note that one of the first symptoms recalled by clients in late childhood is nervousness, with panic not appearing until early adulthood. Because it is difficult to find panickers without generalized anxiety, establishing different hereditability rates for panic and generalized anxiety would require at least matching the two groups on severity.

Behavioral geneticists have a lot of work in front of them before we can draw any conclusions one way or the other in this very difficult but potentially rewarding area. It does seem safe to conclude, however, that some aspect of anxiety runs in families and is probably hereditable. But it is not entirely clear just what is inherited. Studies suggesting differential hereditability of panic and generalized anxiety have not controlled for severity—which influences the hereditability of any human trait in a very powerful way. Therefore, it does not seem possible to say that specific anxiety symptoms are inherited differentially. Rather, the best evidence indicates that what is inherited is a vulnerability to develop an anxiety disorder, because even in studies suggesting a strong genetic contribution, no simple or clear mode of genetic transmission is apparent. In these studies, more of the variance seems to be accounted for by environmental influences than by genetic influences (Crowe et al., 1983, Torgerson, 1983a).

But what exactly is this vulnerability? The strongest evidence suggests that it is a labile or overly responsive autonomic nervous system (Barlow, 1988). Eysenck (1967) makes a strong case for this as the underlying biological vulnerability predisposing the development of a clinical anxiety syndrome under the right combination of environmental and psychological conditions. Even stronger evidence is provided by twin studies on the hereditability of specific autonomic nervous system traits. For example, both Hume (1973) and Lader and Wing (1966) showed that habituation of the galvanic skin response (GSR), as well as pulse rate and number of spontaneous fluctuations in GSR, seem to be genetically determined. As McGuffin and Reich (1984) suggest, these psychophysiological characteristics may well reflect the substrate on which are based both the personality trait of emotionality and the clinical anxiety disorders.

Finally, it just does not make sense at this time to conclude that a specific clinical anxiety symptom (whether it be an obsessional thought, a panic attack, or a phobia of enclosed spaces) would be directly inherited as one intact behavioral and emotional response set in the same sort of simple Mendelian mode as hair and eye color. The demonstrated psychosocial influence on the formation of these behavioral and emotional patterns almost surely points to a complex biopsychosocial model of the development of panic and anxiety. In fact, there is no psychiatric or emotional disorder for which a classical Mendelian mode of single-gene heredity seems applicable.

Even for most of the major psychotic disorders where suggestions of genetic links have long been established, almost all investigators, including geneticists, conclude that an underlying vulnerability exists that interacts with a variety of psychological and social factors to produce the disorder (McGuffin & Reich, 1984; Tsaung & Vandermey, 1980). At most, geneticists suggest that a "polygenic multifactorial" model might be appropriate. That is, the underlying genetically determined vulnerability might be normally distributed across the population through the additive effect of many genes (polygenes), but environmental factors also account for a necessary contribution (multifactorial). A new model or theory of anxiety and panic based on both biological and psychological vulnerability is outlined briefly in Chapter 2 and in full detail elsewhere (Barlow, 1988).

In summary, neither the limited evidence from differential treatment response studies (either pharmacological or psychological) nor the more robust and potentially more important evidence from neurobiological or genetic studies suggest anything unique about panic at this point in time. Of course, new data are always appearing and if anything distinctive about panic is found from these areas of inquiry, it would most likely emerge from detailed studies of neurotransmitter receptor systems.

Evidence from Panic Phenomenology

Despite the relatively weak evidence provided by these approaches, a more straightforward method, often overlooked, provides more convincing evidence on the uniqueness of panic that may highlight what is essentially important about panic. This approach examines panic directly and compares it phenomenologically to general anxiety. For example, Taylor et al. (1896) were able to obtain physiological data on episodes of panic and generalized anxiety by ambulatory monitoring during day-to-day activities. Heart rate remained relatively stable during periods of intense anticipatory anxiety and was generally much lower than during panic episodes. Heart rate averaged 89.2 BPM during anticipatory anxiety as compared to 108.2 BPM during panic. But both episodes of anticipatory and panic anxiety were rated subjectively as equally intense! A similar pattern of results was observed by Freedman, Ianni, Ettedgui, and Puthezhath (1985), who compared heart rate recorded during panic attacks and during states of anxiety that were matched in terms of intensity but were not labeled as panic. The latter, which presumably represented periods of anticipatory or generalized anxiety, were not characterized by heart rate elevation.

However, even physiological comparisons involving panic episodes do not adequately rule out the possibility that panic is simply a severe level of generalized anxiety. It is well established that the response systems of anxiety can be discordant at any given time, so that intensity can vary somewhat independently on subjective and physiological measures. For this reason, panic can be reported, on occasion, in the absence of intense physiological arousal (e.g., Taylor et al., 1986).

Other lines of evidence have compared panic subjects with those who have generalized anxiety disorder (GAD), finding higher physiological responsivity both at rest and during certain tasks (Barlow, Cohen, *et al.*, 1984; Liebowitz *et al.*, 1985; Lum, 1976; Rapee, 1986). These differences also show up in higher somatic scores for panickers on questionnaires (Anderson, Noyes, & Crowe, 1984; Barlow, Cohen, *et al.*, 1984; Hoehn-Saric, 1981).

In general, then, panic seems to present somewhat differently and can be identified separately from intense generalized anxiety on measures of phasic response, tonic response, and questionnaire measures. But, there is one other phenomenological feature of panic that may, in fact, be crucial. This feature of panic is best represented by data presented in Figures 1-1 and 1-2, illustrating the sudden overwhelming surge of anxiety experienced both physiologically and subjectively that reaches a peak in several minutes. While the definition in DSM-III-R specifies 10 minutes, one can see that the surge presented in Figures 1-1 and 1-2 reached a peak in closer to 2 minutes (Cohen *et al.*, 1985).

Now we have fascinating evidence supporting what we have known clinically for some time. Many patients become "apprehensive" about the possibility of having an unexpected or uncued panic attack. This suggests a functional relationship between these two phenomenological events that may differ depending on a variety of parameters. For example, Rachman and Levitt (1985) examined the differential consequences of expected and unexpected panics in a setting where cues for panic were readily available—specifically, a small enclosed space used to assess claustrophobia. Volunteers with moderate to severe claustrophobia were subjected to 238 trials of enclosure in a small dark room. Sixty-seven episodes of panic were experienced by 13 claustrophobics. Of those, 50 were expected and correctly predicted whereas 17 were unexpected. Expected panics were not followed by any changes in feelings of safety or anticipatory anxiety preceding subsequent trials (although it did not influence the probability of panic or the actual fear that was experienced during subsequent trials).

Therefore, what might be important about panic are the overwhelming suddenness or intensity of the event, and whether or not the attack is expected. With this phenomenological difference and the evidence for a functional relationship between anxious apprehension and panic, it may not be necessary to establish underlying biological markers or specific genetic contributions before saying that panic is unique. It may be enough to say that panic is unique because it is experienced as unique by the patient. It is experienced this way because of the sudden surge of emotion and the potentially unexpected nature of the event. In this respect, whether this is simply anxiety at a higher intensity or whether it is essentially a different biological event, its uniqueness is established and we need to attend to the functional implications of this uniqueness.

Do All Panics Have Cues?

Another feature of panic we have discussed in some detail elsewhere concerns the ubiquity of this phenomenon (Barlow, 1988; Barlow & Craske, 1988; Barlow et al., 1985). Basically, these data suggest that panic is not limited to the panic disorders but is found across a wide variety of anxiety and affective disorders. For example, estimates of panic in depressed populations range from 30 to 80% or more (Breier, Charney, & Heninger, 1985; Leckman, Weissman, Merikangas, Pauls, Prusoff, 1983; Pariser, Jones, Pinta, Young, & Fontana, 1979; Benshoof, 1987). Generally, very few differences emerge among different types of panic termed "situational," "spontaneous," or "cued." Cued panics, of course, would refer to the type of panic experienced by simple phobics. That is, if one has a spider phobia, one might reliably panic in the presence (cue) of spiders (see Barlow et al., 1985). Thus, the major difference among various types of panic may be whether the client can identify a cue for the panic. A variety of evidence from laboratory provocation studies and clinical observation suggests that panics for which the individual cannot identify a cue may be preceded by internal physiological disequilibrium of one sort or another (Barlow, 1988).

It is possible that the inability to identify consistent cues is due to inadequate measurement of panic. Most clinicians and researchers to date have simply asked the client to recall panic attacks occurring during the previous week (or longer time period). At the same time, these clients are asked to recall antecedents of these attacks. From a psychological measurement perspective, a more satisfactory procedure would involve prospective self-monitoring of panic so that antecedents or cues can be recorded at the time of the panic over a period of days or weeks.

For example, a depressed client presented as an agoraphobic at our clinic with reports of panic associated with leaving the house, going shopping, and so on. A closer prospective analysis revealed that these panic attacks were triggered by having to make a decision, however small (e.g. making out a grocery list, whether to go to a friend's house). The cues for these panics, then, were consistent with a diagnosis of major depression, which raises interesting questions about the relationship of depression and panic (Barlow, 1988). There is increasing evidence that cues for "spontaneous" panic in agoraphobics and clients with panic disorder are usually associated with mild exercise, sexual relations, sudden temperature changes, stress, or other cues that alter physiological functioning in some discernible way, albeit out of the client's immediate awareness. These physiological changes may signal anxiety much as a phobic object or situation signals intense anxiety or panic in situational panics.

Beck (1988), for example, reported the experience of panic after the following kinds of events: fast consumption of a heavy meal, running up stairs, standing suddenly from a seated position, lifting a heavy object, relaxing, dozing, moving quickly from a hot to a cold area, and so on. More recently, we have explored the phenomenon of relaxation-induced panics (Adler, Craske, & Barlow, 1987). This issue arises again when we consider nocturnal panics in the following subsection.

Early descriptions of effort syndrome referred to emotional reactions during or after exercise (e.g., Cohen & White, 1950). Today, effort syndrome would almost certainly be diagnosed as panic disorder. It is also conceivable that the strong loss-of-control element in unexpected panic derives from the inability to readily explain the panic episode. That is, in the absence of cognizance of panic antecedents, an obvious attribution is the loss of control over one's bodily function, as opposed to an anxiety reaction to a specific situation.

Nocturnal Panic

Perhaps the purest example of spontaneous panic is the phenomenon of nocturnal panic. We assessed the characteristics of nocturnal panic in a group of individuals who presented for treatment at the Phobia and Anxiety Disorders Clinic. These people answered affirmatively to the question "Are there times when you awake from sleep in a panic?" They were then questioned specifically about the duration of these attacks, the amount of sleep before onset of panic, the symptom intensity, and the differences between nocturnal and day panics.

The majority of nocturnal panics occurred within 1 to 4 hours of sleep onset (especially between the second and third hours), the time during which slow-wave sleep is most prevalent. Similarly, Taylor et al. (1986) noted that the panics they recorded on a 24-hour basis occurred most frequently between the hours of 1:30 A.M. and 3:00 A.M. Slow-wave sleep tends to be associated with reduced eye movements, lowered blood pressure, and reduced heart rate and respiration.

These are also the common characteristics of wakeful relaxation. It is therefore tempting to make a connection between nocturnal panic and relaxation-induced panic (Cohen et al., 1985). Relaxation is known to be associated with cognitive, physiological, or sensory side effects that may be perceived as unpleasant (Heide & Borkovec, 1984). For example, a person may become alarmed by a decreasing heart rate that occurs during relaxation, a cue to which the panic-prone patient is very sensitive and which may therefore trigger a panic attack. Similarly, during sleep, an individual may be oblivious to his/her environment but remain attuned to personally significant stimuli. For example, a mother could be undisturbed by the noise of a loud truck driving past her house but may awaken to the sound of her baby crying.

Hauri, Friedman, Ravaris, and Fisher (1985) were able to record five nocturnal panics in their sleep laboratory from a group of agoraphobics with panic attacks. They noted that the panics tended to occur in non-rapid-eye-movement (REM) sleep, although occasionally an attack occurred during REM sleep. Non-REM sleep is associated with occasional violent muscular twitches. The agoraphobics were found to spend a greater number of minutes in delta or slow-wave sleep and to exhibit more large movements during sleep in comparison both to a normal group and to a group of psychophysiological insomniacs. It is possible that muscular movements served as cues that precipitated the elevation in physiological activation that preceded awakening in this group of clients.

Approximately 25% of a consecutive series of panickers and agoraphobics with panic attacks who presented at our Phobia and Anxiety Disorders Clinic reported the experience of at least one nocturnal panic attack. Of those, 43% reported that their first symptom upon awakening was cognitive, such as fear of losing control, dying, or going crazy, whereas 57% reported an initial somatic symptom. Fifty-four percent reported that their nocturnal panics were more severe than their daytime panics, 25% said they were less severe, and 21% said they were of equal severity. In terms of symptom frequency, 46% reported that they experienced more symptoms at night, 21% reported fewer symptoms at night, and 33% reported an equal number of symptoms. Nocturnal panic lasted, on average, 24.6 minutes, with a range of 1 to 180 minutes. Eighteen subjects were questioned in detail concerning the occurrence and severity of each DSM-III-R panic symptom during the most recent nocturnal panic. The frequency with which each symptom was cited by the members of the sample is shown in Table 1-3. The symptoms reported with the greatest frequency were strong, rapid, or irregular heartbeat; shortness of breath; hot and/or cold flashes; choking or smothering sensations; trembling; and fear of dying. Also listed in Table 1-3 are mean severity ratings of the symptoms. Difficulty breathing, fear of dying, heart palpitations, and nausea are the most intensely experienced symptoms. Of interest is the finding that shortness of breath is also one of the most frequently and intensely experienced symptoms during that sample's daytime panics, a pattern that differentiates them somewhat from a representative sample of typical panickers (see Table 1-3).

Nocturnal panic attacks could possibly result from sleep apnea. "Sleep apnea" refers to a pause or complete cessation of breathing: "People with such apneas typically go through a repeating cycle of sleep apnea, arousal, resumption of breathing, and sleep once again" (Van Oot, Lane, & Borkovec, 1984, p. 711). The prominence of the reported shortness of breath symptom would certainly suggest sleep apnea. However, two factors suggest otherwise. First, there was no evidence of obesity in our sample of nocturnal panickers (a characteristic that seems to be a necessary precondition for most cases of sleep apnea). Second, the concentration of nocturnal panic during the first 4 hours of the sleep cycle is not consistent with the repeating pattern of sleep apnea.

TABLE 1-3. Number, Percentage, and Average Severity for Those Subjects Reporting Each of the DSM-III-R Panic Symptoms

| Symptom | Nocturnal panickers ($N = 18$) | | | | | | Panickers without nocturnal panic ($N = 46$) | | |
| | Nocturnal | | | Daytime | | | | | |
	Number	%	Mean severity[a]	Number	%	Mean severity[a]	Number	%	Mean severity[a]
Dyspnea	12	67%	2.42	13	72%	2.15	23	50%	2.09
Palpitations	17	94%	2.29	13	72%	2.06	37	80%	2.54
Chest pain	6	33%	1.33	9	50%	1.56	15	33%	1.73
Choking	11	61%	1.90	11	61%	2.00	15	33%	1.73
Nausea	3	17%	2.33	10	56%	2.00	20	43%	2.10
Dizziness	6	33%	1.67	13	72%	2.15	35	76%	2.20
Feeling of unreality	10	56%	1.33	11	61%	1.73	30	65%	2.20
Paresthesias	5	28%	1.60	10	56%	2.00	21	46%	1.91
Hot or cold flashes	12	67%	1.67	14	78%	1.64	35	76%	2.09
Sweating	10	56%	2.00	13	72%	1.62	26	57%	2.08
Faintness	4	22%	2.00	11	61%	1.55	24	52%	2.13
Trembling	11	61%	1.73	14	78%	1.93	29	63%	2.28
Fear of dying	11	61%	2.45	11	61%	2.09	21	46%	2.48
Fear of going crazy or losing control	7	39%	1.98	12	67%	2.17	23	50%	2.52

Note. Reprinted with permission from: Barlow, D. H., & Craske, M. G. The phenomenology of panic. In S. Rachman & J. D. Maser (Eds.), Panic: Psychological perspectives, 1988. Copyright 1988 by Lawrence Erlbaum Associates.

[a]On a scale of 0 to 8.

Several changes in internal state that occur during different phases of the sleep cycle could serve as triggers for a panic-prone person:

- Reduced heart rate and respiration during slow-wave and deep sleep, as would occur in the case of deep relaxation.
- Erratic breathing patterns that occur during REM sleep.
- Major muscular twitches that occur during delta or slow-wave sleep.

Although nocturnal panic attacks could be considered the purest example of spontaneous panic, even there it seems possible to identify cues for the panic.

Descriptors of Panic

The phenomenon of panic has accumulated many descriptors and qualifiers: spontaneous, situational, predicted, major, minor, and so forth. In our view, the current evidence suggests that panic can best be categorized by the use of the terms "expected" and "cued" and their antonyms, as presented in Table 1-4. For example, claustrophobics report panicking in small enclosed places. This, then, is their reported "cue" for panic, a cue readily understood by the patient. However, as Rachman and Levitt (1985) have clearly demonstrated, claustrophobics may either expect or not expect to have a panic at a given time when entering a small enclosed place. Similarly, agoraphobics may identify a variety of cues for their panics, including shopping malls, crowded spaces, but they may also have panics in the absence of any of these cues—for example, when they are in a safe place or with a safe person. Because identifiable cues preceding panic are in many cases cognitive (Barlow et al., 1985), the term "cue" seems preferable to the term "situational."

TABLE 1-4. Panic Qualifiers

	Expected	Unexpected
Cued		
Uncued		

Clinicians are also well aware that many patients who have panic disorder with or without agoraphobia report expectations of panic in the absence of any identifiable cues. Most often this occurs when agoraphobics awaken and report that they are going to have a "bad day," which means they expect to experience a number of panics. Thus, cued panics can be either expected or unexpected and uncued panics can also be either expected or unexpected. Naturally, the term "cued" is phenomenological in that it refers only to the individual's perception of the presence of a discriminated cue and not to the actual presence of a cue. At this time, all clinical investigators believe that there are clear antecedents, either biological or psychological, for all panic attacks. Nevertheless, whether the person perceives a cue or not (regardless of the actual existence of the cue) has important implications for symptom development, particularly in terms of the development of avoidance behavior. That is, clients tend to avoid a cue perceived to be associated with panic. For these reasons, we begin utilizing the terms "cued" and "expected" throughout the remainder of this book.

Prevalence of Panic

Studies from around the world are converging to suggest that occasional panic attacks occur relatively frequently in the general population. The first study to suggest this was reported by Norton, Harrison, Hauch, and Rhodes (1985), who administered questionnaires to 186 presumably normal young adults. Fully 34.4% of these subjects reported having had one or more panic attacks in the previous year. The percentage reporting more frequent attacks during the previous year decreases markedly. For example, of this 34.4%, 17.2% reported two or more attacks in the past year, 11.3% reported three to four panic attacks, while 6% reported five or more attacks in the past year. While 17.2% reported experiencing one panic attack in the previous 3 weeks, 4.8% (or nine subjects) reported two panic attacks in the previous week, a frequency that would meet DSM-III criteria for panic disorder. In addition, 2.1% (four subjects) reported avoiding some activities or situations because of panic attacks.

One interesting facet of these data is that the number reporting panic attacks that would meet clinical criteria is very close to, and even a little bit less than, what we might expect based on recent epidemiologic investigations (reviewed in the following passages; Myers et al., 1984). This fact, as well as subsequent replication, lends credence to these data. These nonclinical panickers also reported significantly more depression, anxiety, and phobic anxiety on the well-known and often-used Hopkins

Symptom Checklist—90 (Derogatis, Lipman, & Covi, 1973) than those who had never panicked.

It is also interesting to observe that these nonclinical panickers seem to experience fewer symptoms and less-severe symptoms during their panics than panic patients. For example, the infrequent panickers experienced an average of 8 symptoms, whereas the patients reported in Table 1-2 reported 10 or more symptoms. In addition, patients studied by Barlow *et al.* (1985) reported average symptom severity ratings of 1.55 on a scale of 0 to 8, while the nonclinical panickers' average symptom severity score was 1.15. Of course, as Norton, Dorward, and Cox (1986) suggest, it may be that some of these persons will progress into full-blown panic disorder and increase the number of symptoms they report, as well as their ratings of symptom severity.

While assessment of the presence or absence of panic attacks by questionnaire can be justifiably criticized, more careful assessment of 24 of these nonclinical subjects (who reported panic by structured interview) revealed that 22 met DSM-III criteria for panic attacks (but not necessarily panic disorder). The remaining two subjects actually reported experiencing intense nonpanic anxiety (Harrison, 1985). This finding also supports the validity of these data.

In a cross-validation study reported by Norton *et al.* (1986), 256 subjects completed a variety of questionnaires, including a more sophisticated questionnaire than was used in the first study. This questionnaire assessed not only the presence or absence of panic attacks, but also severity, temporal factors associated with the attacks, and whether the attacks were predictable or unpredictable, and so on. Once again, panickers scored significantly higher than nonpanickers on general anxiety and depression as measured by a number of scales, such as the State–Trait Anxiety Inventory, the Beck Depression Inventory, as well as anxiety and depression subscales of the Profile of Mood States. Closely replicating the first study, 35.9% (or 92 subjects) reported experiencing one or more panic attacks in the previous year, with 22.6% experiencing a panic attack within the previous 3 weeks. Other data are also comparable to the first report, and both sets of data are presented in Table 1-5.

New information provided in this replication ascertains the situations in which nonclinical panickers reported experiencing panic attacks. Situations most frequently associated with panic attacks were public speaking, mentioned by 55.2% of all panickers; interpersonal conflict, 46.6%; periods of high stress, 54.5%; and tests and exams, 77.3%. Further, 27.6% of the subjects reported experiencing panic attacks totally out of the blue or, in other words, without any identifiable precipitant whatsoever. In addition, 13.8% reported panics during sleep, and 8.6%

TABLE 1-5. Panic in the Normal Population

Number of panic attacks	1985 ($N = 186$)	1986 ($N = 256$)
1 or more in last year	34.4%	35.9%
Last year		
1–2	17.2%	
3–4	11.3%	
5 or more	6.0%	
Last 3 weeks		
1	17.2%	12.5%
2	4.8%	7.0%
3 or more	2.1%	3.1%

Note. Adapted from Norton et al. (1985, 1986).

during relaxation. The number and severity of symptoms were similar to the earlier study.

The investigators also compared subjects with predictable (cued, expected) versus unpredictable (uncued, unexpected) panics. As with data for clinical panickers (Barlow et al., 1985), those with uncued, unpredictable, unexpected attacks experienced more panic attacks and rated two symptoms—tachycardia and unreality—as being somewhat more severe than those with predictable (cued and expected) attacks. Similar data on the prevalence of panic in the general population have recently been reported from Great Britain (Gerald M. Klerman, personal communication, 1986).

Another factor that builds confidence in the validity of these findings is data on the aggregation of panic and other psychopathology in the families of nonclinical infrequent panickers. For example, Norton et al. (1986) found that a significantly greater proportion of panickers than nonpanickers reported fathers, mothers, brothers, and sisters who had had panic attacks. These findings are particularly strong because the results were statistically significant for each class of relatives, rather than just in the aggregate. These data resemble the aforementioned results demonstrating a high familial aggregation of panic in the families of patients (Barlow, 1988). For example, Crowe et al. (1983) found that 25% of first-order relatives of panic disorder patients also met DSM-III criteria for panic disorder. An additional 30% experienced infrequent panic attacks. In Norton et al. (1986), approximately 30% of first-order relatives were reported to experience panic. The data from Crowe et al. also attest to the seemingly high prevalence of panic in the population at large.

Prevalence of Panic Disorder

Millions of individuals each year seek help for what is broadly construed as anxiety or nervousness. Statistics compiled from the offices of front-line primary care practitioners startle even the most jaded experts in the area. In Virginia, investigators surveying the reasons patients sought out their local physicians found that hypertension, cuts and bruises, and sore throats rank right behind a general medical check-up as the most common reason motivating a visit (Marsland, Woods, & Mayo, 1976). Close behind these common maladies was "anxiety," which even ranked ahead of bad colds or bronchitis. Most likely, unexpected panic attacks play a large role in motivating these visits.

Who are these people? Does everyone who seeks out a local physician or health care practitioner complaining of "anxiety" or "nerves" really suffer from anxiety or panic? Does everyone who takes minor tranquilizers have a clearly defined anxiety disorder? Most clinicians and investigators would guess that these millions of individuals do not present with clearly identifiable anxiety disorders but rather with some vague combination of stress, adjustment to difficult family or work situations, or other temporary problems such as difficulty sleeping. For years it was impossible to actually ascertain the number of these individuals presenting with anxiety disorders. Since the mid-1980s, epidemiologists have begun to undertake this arduous task, culminating in the most ambitious studies of the prevalence of anxiety disorders ever undertaken.

Two very important developments have made more sophisticated and wide-ranging efforts possible. First, diagnostic criteria for specific anxiety disorders were specified in much more detail such that two different interviewers could agree whether a given individual had a specific anxiety disorder or not. Second, structured interviews were devised that ensured that all investigators covered all essential materials in very much the same way when interviewing for the presence of panic (or other) disorders. These developments ensured a much more standardized and objective approach to the question of the frequency of specific disorders in the population. Preliminary data are now available from the National Institute of Mental Health (NIMH)-sponsored Epidemiologic Catchment Area (ECA) Survey, which has been ongoing in five different sites around the country since 1980. The population size in each site is approximately 300,000, and up to 5,000 or more individuals in each site were interviewed using a structured interview by an individual trained to administer this interview.

For our purposes, the data on disorders where unexpected panic plays a prominent role are of particular interest. These disorders, of course, are panic disorder and agoraphobia. Results on these disorders from the first wave of interviews are presented in Table 1-6.

These are startling figures. Among the many mysteries and paradoxes presented in these data, the estimates of the prevalence of agoraphobia in the population have risen from the 0.6% figure in earlier epidemiologic studies (e.g., Agras, Sylvester, & Oliveau, 1969) to between 2.7 and 5.8% in the ECA Survey. Even if one discounts the rather high estimate from Baltimore, this represents almost a fivefold increase in estimates of prevalence. This would indicate, for example, that in the United States alone, between 9 and 15 million individuals suffer from panic disorder with or without agoraphobia. Because agoraphobia with panic is now considered to be a subcategory of panic disorder in DSM-III-R (see below), these figures concern us directly for the purposes of this book even though we do not deal directly with agoraphobic avoidance.

What could account for these startling differences in estimates of prevalence? It may simply be the way the questions were asked. In the Agras et al. (1969) study, very conservative criteria were used, but it seems unlikely that this could account for all of the difference. In the aforementioned ECA Survey, lengthy structured interviews and specific, reliable diagnostic definitions were employed that, when combined with the enormous numbers of people involved, tends to make one more confident in these data. In the time between the two studies, there has also been a substantial increase in awareness of the problem of agoraphobia, although, once again, it is hard to see how this could account for absolute increases in the prevalence of the problem. For now, this discrepancy remains a mystery.

TABLE 1-6. Six-Month Prevalence of DSM-III Anxiety Disorder Diagnoses

	New Haven	Baltimore	St. Louis
Panic (%)			
Male	0.3	0.8	0.7
Female	0.9	1.2	1.0
Total	0.6	1.0	0.9
Agoraphobia (%)			
Male	1.1	3.4	0.9
Female	4.2	7.8	4.3
Total	2.8	5.8	2.7

Note. Adapted from Myers et al. (1984).

Male–Female Ratios

Another startling figure of which we have been aware for some time is evident in the data on agoraphobia. Almost 75% of all agoraphobics are women. This has been a remarkably consistent finding around the world, which in some studies is even more dramatic. For example, Burns and Thorpe (1977) interviewed 963 agoraphobics as part of a national survey throughout the British Isles. Fully 88% of these agoraphobics were women. What could account for this difference?

At least four different hypotheses have attracted varying amounts of attention. Some investigators have assumed that there are just as many male agoraphobics, but that for cultural reasons, it is more acceptable for females to express fear and anxiety. Therefore, more females come for treatment. The ECA data, however, would seem to undermine this hypothesis because population surveys confirm the preponderance of women. A second hypothesis suggests that the differences in prevalence between males and females are real and due to the fact that females have biologically based wider-ranging endocrinological changes that make them more susceptible to panic. A third hypothesis also suggests that the differences are real but once again culturally based in that males are taught to "tough out" or endure their fears, leading to early and more complete extinction of any avoidance behavior when compared to females.

The fourth hypothesis suggests, however, that the numbers with underlying panic attacks are more nearly equal. Only in reactions to panic do differences emerge. That is, females cope with panic by avoiding while males cope by other means, such as self-medicating with alcohol. Now evidence is emerging supporting this hypothesis (Barlow, 1988; Chambless & Mason, 1986). Thus, it seems that the occurrence of panic may be more nearly (but not totally) equal among males and females but that there are culturally determined differences in methods of coping with panic. If this evidence holds up, a substantial proportion of problem drinkers may require attention to an underlying panic disorder as an important component of their treatment program. This issue is addressed next.

Mortality and Substance Abuse

Self-defeating behavior associated with anxiety and panic rarely produces death, but long-term follow-up studies of both inpatients (Coryell, Noyes, & Clancy, 1982) and outpatients (Coryell, Noyes, & House, 1986) have found a greater-than-expected death rate in patients with panic disorder. The excess mortality seems due primarily to two different causes: cardiovascular disease and suicide. In fact, suicide rates in panic patients were equal to or slightly greater than a matched group of patients suffering from depression. Interestingly, excess mortality due to cardiovascular disease was limited to males with panic disorder. Expected death rates for females with panic disorder from cardiovascular disease were normal.

Death by suicide has been associated almost exclusively with depression. The fact that preliminary studies find an equal frequency in patients with anxiety and panic is a frightening discovery. Why would people who are anxious kill themselves? Coryell *et al.* (1986) speculate that patients initially diagnosed with panic disorder may subsequently develop complications of alcoholism or depression. But if alcoholism or depression is a consequence of panic and anxiety, then the long road to suicide begins with anxiety and panic.

A series of investigators suggest that the relationship between substance abuse, particularly alcohol abuse, and anxiety disorders is startlingly high. For example, Quitkin, Rifkin, Kaplan, and Klein (1972) reported, in some detail, on 10 patients with anxiety disorders who also suffered severe complications from drug and alcohol abuse. While this was always a common clinical observation, a study appearing in 1979 by Mullaney and Trippett attracted new attention to this potentially severe complication of anxiety and panic. They discovered that 33% of 102 alcoholics also had severe disabling agoraphobia and/or social phobia. In addition, another 35% had mild versions of the same phobias. Thus, over 60% of a large group of alcoholics who were admitted to an alcoholism treatment unit presented with identifiable anxiety disorders of varying severity.

Smail, Stockwell, Canter, and Hodgson (1984) explored this same question in a particularly systematic and skillful way and found similar, although somewhat less dramatic, results. Specifically, 18% of a group of 60 alcoholics also presented with severe agoraphobia and/or social phobia, with another 35% evidencing mild versions of the same phobia. Once again, over half (53% of this group of alcoholics) had identifiable anxiety disorders. Other more recent studies came to similar conclusions. For example, Chambless, Cherney, Caputo, and Rheinstein (1987) carefully interviewed a group of 75 inpatient alcoholics and ascertained that 40% presented with a lifetime diagnosis of one or more anxiety disorders. Studies using somewhat more conservative criteria also report a rather high range from 25 to 45% of severe alcoholics also presenting with one or more anxiety disorders (Bowen, Cipywnyk, D'Arcy, & Keegan, 1984; Mullan, Gurling, Oppenheim, & Murray, 1986; Powell, Penick, Othmer,

Bingham, & Rice, 1982; Weiss & Rosenberg, 1985). The important suggestion by Quitkin *et al.* (1972) was that patients presenting with substance abuse problems may well be self-medicating anxiety or panic and that any treatment program must target anxiety to be successful during treatment as well as to prevent relapse.

The obvious question is which comes first, the anxiety or the substance abuse. Several investigators have looked at this issue, and the emerging evidence suggests that a complex relationship exists. Retrospective studies indicate that severe anxiety precedes the onset of drinking or substance abuse in most cases (Chambless *et al.*, 1987; Mullaney & Trippett, 1979; Smail *et al.*, 1984). But there are some patients for whom the development of anxiety seems to follow serious substance abuse. Also, periods of abstinence seem to result in a general improvement in fear and anxiety in many patients (e.g., Smail *et al.*, 1984).

There is now direct experimental evidence of a phenomenon reasonably well documented in the field of alcoholism; that is, contrary to myth, alcohol does not necessarily reduce anxiety and fear and may, in fact, worsen it (Thyer & Curtis, 1984). As Smail *et al.* (1984) suggest, severe anxiety and panic disorders may well precede substance abuse in many cases, and the initial use of alcohol or drugs may be primarily for anxiolytic purposes. Nevertheless, once addicted, the alcohol (or drug) may have a deleterious effect on mood, creating a vicious cycle. For this reason, patients with anxiety disorders who are also alcoholic may present with more severe anxiety (Chambless *et al.*, 1987) because of the use of alcohol. Thus, anxiety self-medicated with alcohol results in an ever-increasing downward self-destructive spiral, not only from the effects of alcohol (or drug) addiction, but also from the exacerbating effects of the drugs on the anxiety itself. It may be this complication, along with the resulting development of helplessness and depression, that leads to the increased risk of suicide in patients with anxiety (Coryell *et al.*, 1986).

Summary

Although there is still much to learn about panic and panic disorder, we are now beginning to view panic as a unique emotional event. While only a minority of individuals go on to develop panic disorder, this event results in substantial disability in individuals who experience panic. The pain and suffering associated with panic disorder, and the marked complications that arise from maladaptive attempts to cope with unexpected panic through substance abuse or avoidance, result in enormous personal loss as well as substantial costs to our health care systems. For this reason, attempts to develop effective treatments for panic are essential. But the development of effective treatments depends on a working theoretical model of panic and associated anxious apprehension. A brief outline of a model emerging from emotion theory, as well as derivative treatments, constitutes the next chapter.

2

The Conception and Treatment of Panic

One-Dimensional Models

Our treatment approach to panic is firmly based on an emerging model of panic and anxiety (Barlow, 1988). This model takes into consideration biological, psychological, and social or environmental factors. Each of these factors seems to contribute to emotional disorders where panic is a prominent feature. The purpose of this chapter is to sketch out this model of panic and panic disorder and review briefly derivative psychological treatments as well as existent drug treatments. Preliminary evidence for the effectiveness of the treatment protocol that forms the bulk of this book is presented toward the end of the chapter.

The study of panic is in its infancy. Therefore, it is not surprising that current models of panic tend to be one-dimensional. For example, biological models of panic point to random biological dysregulations resulting in eruptions of emotion that we call panic. In these causal models, the neurobiological eruption can account for all of the symptoms of panic. In this way, panic is a unique event and can be distinguished from generalized anxiety. Speculations on the source of these disruptions range far and wide, across a variety of central and peripheral mechanisms. As this research advances, we are learning a great deal more about the neurobiological basis of anxiety and panic (e.g., Ballenger, 1986; Wambolt & Insel, 1988). Models based on biological dysregulation have received by far the most experimental attention to date.

It would seem logical that a biological dysregulation underlies panic. After all, the very nature of panic as present in panic disorder specifies that there is no readily identifiable antecedent or cue. For this reason, investigators have attempted to identify a biological marker in individuals with panic disorder that would be associated with an underlying biological dysregulation, or at least point in the direction of a biological dysregulation. This research and the leading biological models of panic are reviewed elsewhere (Barlow, 1988). Among the many current possibilities mentioned are deficiencies in alpha-2 receptors, which would tend to cause surges in norepinephrine; abnormalities in the locus ceruleus, with a resulting dysregulation of the modulation of sensory input; or, most recently, heightened central CO_2 sensitivity, which would make individuals susceptible to rapid breathing and feelings of suffocation.

But biological researchers have not yet been able to come up with any specific biological marker or, for that matter, any important neurobiological differences between persons with panic disorder and nonpanickers. Even if a biological dysregulation is discovered, it will be difficult to determine whether this is a cause or effect of the disorder. One factor consistently found in panic disorder is chronic overarousal, which seems a biological marker of sorts. But, chronic overarousal and its as-yet-undiscovered biological underpinnings characterizes almost all anxiety disorders and would not qualify as a specific biological marker for panic. However, it may interact with other variables and contribute to the genesis of panic disorder in a manner suggested in the following passages. For these and other reasons, many leading neurobiological researchers are eschewing one-dimensional biological models of panic in favor of more complex biopsychological models (e.g., Liebowitz, 1986).

An alternative one-dimensional model beginning to receive increased attention is the cognitive model of panic. These developing models are based on the creative theorizing and important clinical innovation of Aaron T. Beck (e.g., Beck & Emery, 1985). In its simplest form, this model assumes that the sharp spiral into panic is due to catastrophic misinterpretations of otherwise normal bodily sensations. Implicit in this theorizing is the notion that nothing particularly unique is occurring in the individual from a neurobiological perspective. For example, mild chest pain experienced after certain types of exercise might be interpreted in a vulnerable individual as an impending heart attack. Individuals developing panic disorder would differ from those who did not only in their tendencies to misinterpret somatic events in a variety of ways. Thus, panic would be considered, by and large, to be a severe form of generalized anxiety.

More recently, sophisticated cognitive theorists (Clark, 1986; Rapee, 1987; Salkovskis, 1988) have suggested that biological disruptions may play a role in some panic attacks. For example, they theorize that there are individual differences in respiratory response to stress. That is, in certain stressful situations, vulnerable individuals will overbreathe, resulting in a hyperventilatory episode. Hyperventilation will then produce a variety of physical sensations. In some individuals, these sensations will be misinterpreted in a catastrophic fashion. The consequence is panic. The cause of panic, then, is not seen as a hyperventilatory episode, but rather the catastrophic misinterpretation of symptoms produced by hyperventilation. Of course, as these authors acknowledge, there are many pathways to panic (Barlow, 1986, 1988), and hyperventilation does not seem in any way a necessary or sufficient condition for the occurrence of panic (Gelder, 1986; Barlow, 1988). This theorizing begins to move away from a one-dimensional cognitive model of panic, but the burden, of course, is placed squarely on cognitive distortion.

A View from Emotion Theory

In another approach developed at length elsewhere (Barlow, 1988), panic is neither a random biological dysregulation nor a cognitive misinterpretation of somatic cues, although both of these factors are present to some extent.

In this view, one cannot understand panic without understanding the nature of anxiety and fear. In turn, one cannot understand anxiety and fear without referring to the accumulated wisdom of emotion theory because panic and anxiety are primarily emotions. In their pathological expressions, they become emotional disorders.

Almost all emotion theorists consider anxiety a loose cognitive-affective structure. Theorists as diverse as Izard (1977), Lang (1985), and Hallam (1985) consider anxiety (and depression) to be a pervasive, diffuse state that may represent either a blend of basic emotions (Izard, 1977) or a rather loose, widespread affective network stored in memory (Lang, 1985). This construct may also have multiple referents. That is, the phenomena that one individual refers to as anxiety may be very different than the referents used by another individual (Hallam, 1985).

In our view (Barlow, 1988), this loose cognitive-affective structure is characterized by a variety of cognitive and behavioral operations not generally considered to be within the purview of emotions. These operations can be organized into a negative-feedback cycle characterized, to varying degrees, both by components of high negative affect and by perceptions that both internal and external events are proceeding in an unpredictable, uncontrollable fashion. This perception of uncontrollability also seems to be accompanied by a disruption or interruption of attention with a shift away from the task at hand to internal, self-evaluative modes. Anxiety, then, may be best characterized as marked apprehension surrounding the possible occurrence of unpleasant or dangerous events in the future; "It could happen again and I might not be able to deal with it." For this reason, the term "anxious apprehension" might refer more precisely to this diffuse future-oriented mood state. Anxiety also implies an effort to cope with difficult situations, and the physiology (arousal) is there to support active attempts at coping when necessary. This contrasts with depression, for example, where the individual seems to have given up. This theory of anxiety is outlined more fully elsewhere (Barlow, 1988).

But, if anxiety is a clinical manifestation of a diffuse cognitive-affective structure spanning a variety of emotional, cognitive, and behavioral operations, then what is fear? Most emotion theorists consider fear as a tightly organized focal, intense emotion that may represent a cohesive or coherent affective structure (Lang, 1985) or perhaps a distinct, primative, basic emotion (Izard, 1977). Indeed, many emotion theorists consider fear to be a primary alarm in response to present danger characterized by high negative affect and arousal. There is no mistaking it for other basic emotions such as sadness. Evidence exists suggesting that the basic emotion of fear is found invariantly across cultures, races, and species, as well as far down the phylogenetic scale.

Creative theorists such as Beck (e.g., Beck & Emery, 1985) have long insisted on considering the functional significance or the evolutionary purpose of behavior in general and of emotions in particular. This has not been difficult with fear. To almost all observers, beginning with Darwin (1872), the alarm of fear has been responsible in large part for the survival of the species. Those individual organisms capable of becoming quickly alarmed, with the accompanying mobilization of the body for fight or flight, survived and won the day while those not so inclined perished. Based on this point of view then, fear is an ancient, probably hard-wired alarm system enabling the organism to respond to emergencies (Cannon, 1929). But, what is the clinical manifestation of fear? In our view, fear is panic and panic is the unadulterated, ancient, hard-wired alarm system we call fear.

When confronted with an immediate threat to our well-being which, quite fortunately, is experienced very seldom these days, we share this reaction with our ancestors who lived in caves. It has been demonstrated again and again that our physical capacities to perform necessary actions are greatly enhanced during fear when our objective is clear. Our objective, of course, is fight or flight. But what if there is no objective?

No cue? No threat? Under these circumstances, the reaction is a false alarm and it is not surprising that it is a devastating experience. If uncued, unexpected panic is a false alarm, then it will be crucial to determine the causes of false alarms. Evidence has begun to accumulate on this issue.

Causes of False Alarms

While many investigators continue to explore immediate causes of false alarms such as biological dysregulation or cognitive distortion, other evidence points to more-distant events that may relate to the later development of panic disorder. Theorizing has centered on two issues: separation anxiety and the experience of stressful life events. By far, the strongest evidence relates to stress.

Stress

A remarkably consistent observation of biological and psychological clinicians and investigators for a number of years has been the extremely high evidence of negative life events preceding the first panic attack in patients later presenting with panic disorder. What makes this more interesting is that few of these patients can identify a precipitating event when asked a question such as "What caused your first panic attack?" However, further systematic questioning about life events reveals that approximately 80% of these patients will describe very clearly a negative life event closely associated with their first panic (Buglass, Clarke, Henderson, Kreitman, & Presley, 1977; Doctor, 1982; Finlay-Jones & Brown, 1981; Mathews, Gelder, & Johnston, 1981; Roth, 1959; Snaith, 1968; Solyom, Beck, Solyom, & Hugel, 1974; Uhde et al., 1985). For example, Shafar (1976) reported precipitating stressors in 83% of her sample, and Sheehan, Sheehan, and Minichiello (1981) reported it in 91% of their large sample.

Typical of these studies and the types of negative life events reported are results from an early series of 58 agoraphobics (53 females and 5 males) from our clinic (Last, Barlow, & O'Brien, 1984). The occurrence of negative life events was assessed by structured clinical interview. Categories of life events and the frequencies with which they were reported are presented in Table 2-1. Of the 58 agoraphobics, 81% reported one or more of these stressful life events, while 19% reported no significant life event prior to the development of agoraphobia. For heuristic purposes, we collapsed life events reported by our clients into conflict events versus endocrine/physiological reactions (see Table 2-1). These two major categories accounted for approximately 91% of the life events reported. Liebowitz and Klein (1979) also reported a large proportion of individuals developing panic attacks after experiencing endocrinological changes. And Klein, in an early survey (1964), noted "endocrine fluctuations" such as those associated with birth, menopause, gynecological surgery, and so forth, as events immediately preceding panic in a subgroup of patients.

Perhaps the best study in this group was also one of the earliest. Roth (1959) found that 96% of a sample of 135 agoraphobics reported some type of background stress preceding the development of their disorder. The stressors of 83% of these patients were categorized as follows: bereavement or a suddenly developing serious illness in a close relative or friend (37%); illness or acute danger to the patient (31%); severance of family ties or acute domestic stress (15%). In an additional 13% of the women, panic began during pregnancy or after childbirth, and was characterized by an abrupt onset shortly after delivery. What makes this study strong is that Roth was the only one to employ a control group. He found that the incidence of identifiable stressors in his agoraphobic patients was significantly greater than that found in 50 control patients suffering from some other form of neurosis, as well as 50

TABLE 2-1. Life Events Occurring Prior to Onset of Agoraphobia

Precipitating events	Frequency ($N = 58$)	%
Interpersonal conflict situations		
Marital/familial	20	34.5%
Death/illness of significant other	9	15.5%
Total	29	50.0%
Endocrine/physiological reactions		
Birth/miscarriage/hysterectomy	17	29.3%
Drug reaction	7	12.1%
Total	24	41.4%
Other		
Major surgery/illness (other than gynecological)	2	3.4%
Stress at work/school	2	3.4%
Move	2	3.4%

Note. Frequencies exceed the number of patients interviewed because many patients reported more than one significant life event occurring prior to their first panic attack. Reprinted with permission of publisher from: Last, C. G., Barlow, D. H., & O'Brien, G. T. Precipitants of agoraphobia: Role of stressful life events. *Psychological Reports*, 1984, *54*, 567–570. Tables 1 and 2.

additional individuals who had recently recovered from a physical illness
but had never suffered a psychiatric disorder. More recently, Roy-Byrne,
Geraci, and Uhde (1986) replicated those findings, comparing panic
disorder patients with healthy controls.

These data, consistent as they are, have led many to assume that
stress plays a major role in the etiology of panic (Mathews *et al.*, 1981;
Margraf *et al.*, 1986; Tearnan, Telch, & Keefe, 1984). But what can we
conclude from these intriguing observations? While the consistency of
these observations attests to the reliability of reports of this relationship,
one cannot escape the fact that these are retrospective reports.

It is also becoming increasingly apparent that stress, defined as
negative life events, seems to be associated with the onset or exacerbation
of any number of physical and psychological disorders. For example,
relationships have been demonstrated between stress and cardiovascular
disease, complications associated with pregnancy and birth, tuberculosis,
multiple sclerosis, diabetes, chronic back pain, and depression, to name
only a few (e.g., Depue, 1979; Flor, Turk, & Birbaumer, 1985; Hammen,
Mayol, deMayo, & Marks, 1986; Lewinsohn, Hoberman, & Rosenbaum,
in press; Lloyd, 1980).

The most common explanation for the effects of stress is the well-
known stress–diathesis model wherein stress precipitates and facilitates a
particular physical or emotional disorder to which the individual is
already predisposed. In the case of psychophysiological stress responses
such as hypertension, ulcers, and so on, the "weak organ" model best
expresses this hypothesis. Essentially (and simplistically) the effects of
stress overactivates one's (physiological) system until the weakest part of
the system breaks down. This weakness might be constitutional or a
result of earlier traumatic processes (Selye, 1976).

Within psychological disorders, such as panic disorder, the hypothetical process is a little less clear due to the aforementioned methodological difficulties. Nevertheless, it is possible that a number of individuals are vulnerable to panicking during periods of stress, just as others are
vulnerable to other types of disorders such as headaches or ulcers.

But a common finding across all disorders studied is that even acute
stress, usually defined as a negative life event, correlates only modestly
with psychopathology. That is, while there may be a clear association, as
it certainly seems there is with panic, a large number of people, even if
prone to a disorder, experience similar life events without developing
panic or some alternative disorder. Most usually it is assumed that
moderating variables such as certain cognitive and personality variables,
as well as social support, diminish the effects of stress (e.g., Depue &
Monroe, 1986; Sarason & Sarason, 1981).

Thus, a variety of evidence indicates that certain individuals susceptible to stress produced by negative life events because of constitutional
factors, relatively low social support, and/or some combination of personality and cognitive dispositions, react to negative life events in much
the same way they might react to physical threats from wild animals or
snakes. That is, they evidence a basic hard-wired fear response much as
they would when confronted with any other threat to their well-being.
Because the fear response is not temporally associated within hours with
the negative life event, the individual is unable to specify an antecedent to
the fear or a cause. Indeed there is no antecedent that would require an
immediate alarm reaction with all of its associated action tendencies of
fight or flight. For that reason, the alarm is false. Of course, the false
alarm does not directly follow the stressful event. Other factors, both
biological and cognitive, undoubtedly contribute to proneness to false
alarms under conditions of stress.

If the stress–diathesis model of false alarms and panic is correct,
then one would predict that infrequent nonclinical panickers would
continue having occasional false alarms of varying severity, depending on
their vulnerability to false alarms, their threshold for stressful events they
may be experiencing, moderating variables, and, among other things, the
intensity and frequency of negative life events. But for a minority of
individuals for whom circumstances line up correctly, the relationship
does not stay as simple as this. The overwhelming experience of panic in
these individuals seems to ensure that some learning will take place,
which markedly affects the subsequent course of false alarms.

The Etiology of Phobia and Panic Disorder

With this in mind, we can now consider how false alarms might be
learned and the implication for the etiology of phobia and panic disorder.
For years, investigators have searched the histories of phobic individuals
for signs of traumatic conditioning. The primary finding is that most
phobics cannot recall a traumatic conditioning event to account for the
development of their fear or phobia. It is also clear that many fears and
some phobias are acquired vicariously (Murray & Foote, 1979; Rimm,
Janda, Lancaster, Nahl, & Dittmar, 1977). But more recent information
suggests that false alarms may play a major role.

For example, McNally and Steketee (1985) interviewed 22 outpatients presenting for treatment with animal phobias. When questioned
about etiology, most (15) of these patients could not remember what
happened. Of the remaining 7 cases, 5 did have a frightening encounter

with an animal whereas 2 seemed to acquire their fear through instructional or vicarious modes. Nevertheless, what they all dreaded now was not that the animal they feared would attack them—rather, they were afraid they would panic and suffer the consequences of panic following an unavoidable encounter with the animal.

Munjack (1984), in a very interesting retrospective analysis, questioned a more common type of simple phobia about the etiology of fear: patients with a fear of driving. Of his 30 subjects, a few (20%) reported some traumatic incident while driving that seemed to lead to their fears, such as a collision. But almost half reported no such incident. Rather, they noted that suddenly for no apparent reason they panicked while driving and since then had been unable to drive on freeways. While these patients presented with a fear of driving, what actually seems to make them anxious, much as with McNally and Steketee's (1985) patients, is the possibility of having another panic attack. Even in the remaining patients where the etiology was not clear, it seems possible that experiences similar to panic or limited symptom attacks might have played a role.

It is entirely possible then, that a few simple phobics experience an alarm reaction in response to a realistic threat to their well-being, which then becomes associated with the same or similar objects or situations. Being attacked by a dog might be an example. However, many simple phobics experience a false alarm. This false alarm is of such intensity that learning also occurs. Specifically, false alarms become strongly associated with the object or situations that set the occasion for the first false alarm. This association would represent basic emotional learning (conditioned emotional response) rather than a simple misinterpretation, although catastrophic misinterpretations would certainly be present if one searched for them. In this model, the individual would evidence anxiety in the presence of the object or situation (or similar objects or situations), which set the occasion for the first false alarm. But anxiety would occur primarily over the possibility of having another (unpredictable) false alarm in the presence of the cues that signal the possibility of this alarm.

The implications of this model for simple phobics are clear. An actual traumatic event (true alarm) involving the phobic object or situation would not be necessary. All that would be required would be a false alarm in the presence of a previously benign object or situation to ensure that a learned alarm might occur the next time the object or situation were encountered. Of course, this would not be a random event. For example, phobic development is more likely if the object or situation were "prepared" in an evolutionary sense (Seligman, 1971; Öhman, Dimberg, & Öst, 1985). That is, we are more likely to develop fear of snakes than electrical outlets because the propensity to develop this fear served our ancestors well. But development of much phobic behavior, in our view, is due to inadvertent interference with the powerful escapist action tendencies associated with our alarm reaction. Hence the common theme of feeling trapped runs through many phobic situations, as we shall see.

False Alarms and Panic Disorder

But what of patients with panic disorder? The majority of these individuals are unable to report a clearly demarcated cue for their alarms (such as small animals, planes, or public speaking), although agoraphobics often report a series of diffuse situations of which they are wary. It is possible that the major difference between agoraphobics and other phobics may be whether they have associated their false alarm with a specific cue or not. What is learned in this case? To understand this more fully, one has to consider an important but little known line of research conducted by Russian investigators.

For years, Russian investigators conducted a series of experiments demonstrating that fear could be conditioned to internal physiological stimuli, which came to be known as "interoceptive" stimuli (Razran, 1961). To take one example typical of this line of research, the colon of a dog was slightly stimulated (conditioned stimulus) at the same time that an electric shock was administered to the dog. As a result of this conditioning procedure, the dog began to evidence signs of intense anxiety during the natural passage of feces. The Russians demonstrated that this type of learning was particularly resistant to extinction. That is, it would persist indefinitely despite repeated physiological sensations in the absence of the original unconditioned stimulus (shock).

The clear implication is that it is possible to learn an association between internal cues and false alarms and that these internal cues then serve the same function for patients with panic disorder with or without agoraphobia that external cues do for simple phobics. That is, they signal the possibility of another false alarm.

The association of false alarms with internal or external cues results in the phenomenon of learned alarms. Furthermore, a characteristic of any learned response is that it need not fully replicate its unlearned counterpart. For example, only limited fear propositions present in a given context might elicit one part of the emotion (Lang, 1985). Thus, learned alarms may be only partial responses, such as cognitive representations without the marked physiological component of alarms. *In vivo* monitoring of learned alarms supports this contention (Taylor *et al.*, 1986).

One clear consequence of this learning in those individuals who go on to develop anxiety and become phobic is the rapid development of acute sensitivity and vigilance concerning the newly acquired phobic cues. Someone recently bitten by a dog will quickly become acutely sensitive to any signs of dogs and this vigilance will extend to unfamiliar areas where dogs might be roaming free. Someone experiencing an alarm (or a false alarm) in an elevator will become acutely aware of any plans in the immediate future that might require entry into an elevator. And someone who has learned to associate interoceptive cues with false alarms will become acutely sensitive to and vigilant of specific somatic cues associated with this alarm.

It is also interesting to consider, in this regard, the minority of panic patients who can clearly cite an unfavorable experience with drugs such as anesthesia or cocaine, or a first experience with marijuana as the setting event for their first panic (e.g., Aronson & Craig, 1986). Here, the trigger in terms of a temporally associated event seems clear, and anesthesia and marijuana are avoided. But a full panic disorder syndrome also develops, including marked sensitivity to a variety of somatic cues and repeated panic attacks in the absence of external cues. Once again this would seem to reflect interoceptive conditioning.

Evidence that people presenting with panic disorder fear interoceptive cues is accumulating along several fronts (e.g., Rapee, 1986; van den Hout, van der Molen, Griez, & Lousberg, 1987). This accounts for the consistent clinical observation of the extreme sensitivity to somatic cues in panic patients. Data from studies provoking panic in the laboratory as well as the interesting phenomenon of nocturnal panic support this model (Barlow, 1988; Barlow & Craske, 1988). Of course, if one is trapped in a situation where no exit is possible while experiencing the full effects of the false alarm, it is more likely that attention will be directed toward this trapped situation that prevents the powerful action tendency of escape (flight). Common examples include planes or other means of public transportation; dentist or hairdresser chairs where it is difficult to suddenly get up and leave; or public places like churches where a quick exit might prove embarrassing. This prevention of the presumably hardwired action tendency of escape (flight) may be an ethological contribution to the development of phobic behavior.

Alarms and Anxiety

One final link in the etiologic chain derives from the fascinating issue of who develops clinical disorders associated with false or learned alarms and who does not. As we have seen (Norton et al., 1985, 1986), many more people seem to experience alarms than present with clinical disorders. Infrequent panickers seem to account for a large percentage of the population (over 30%). At present, the difference between those who develop full-blown clinical syndromes and those who do not is largely speculative because we know so little about infrequent panickers. For example, nonclinical panickers with occasional alarms seem to experience them much less frequently, although a small minority were experiencing as many as three in a 3-week period and yet had evidently not considered seeking help. These subjects also experienced their alarms much less intensely.

It is possible, of course, particularly among those who were experiencing more frequent panics, that these would develop further in intensity and frequency to the point where a full-blown panic disorder would develop. However, another possibility is that they simply did not fear these alarms or, more accurately, they were not apprehensively anxious about them. What could account for this?

One possibility is that the alarms simply were not of sufficient intensity to elicit a negative affective response. But, another (more likely) possibility is that people who develop full-blown panic or phobic disorders are specifically susceptible to this type of learning (becoming anxious) due to a combination of individual biological and psychological factors or a combination of the two. Among these factors could be baseline levels of arousal, perceptions of unpredictability and uncontrollability of the alarms or other negative events, poor coping skills, lack of social support, and so forth. In other words, if this alarm calls forth a variety of anxious propositions in Lang's (1985) sense concerning perceptions of unpredictability, uncontrollability, increased arousal surrounding the alarm and a shift of attention to internal self-evaluative modes, then it is possible that the conditions will be ripe for the development of an emotional disorder.

If, on the other hand, one does not experience unpredictability or loss of control from this event, one might, as a consequence, attribute it to predictable events of the moment (something I ate; a fight with my boss). In this case, one would not experience an internal self-evaluative shift in attention, and the false alarm would be just that. Life would then go on as before, with perhaps an occasional rather mild false alarm reappearing from time to time under stressful conditions. In other words, to develop panic disorder, one must be susceptible to developing anxiety or apprehension over the possibility of subsequent alarms or other negative events. Thus, the importance of the loose cognitive-affective structure of anxiety mentioned in the beginning of the chapter becomes apparent.

The development of anxiety, in turn, depends upon specific vulnera-
bilities that are based on both general neurobiological and specific early
learning (psychological) experiences. The cognitive distortions that one
so often sees in panic disorders would then be simply one part of the
diffuse cognitive-affective structure we call "anxiety." This theory of
anxiety and panic is fully elaborated elsewhere (Barlow, 1988). Thus, the
occurrence of false alarms and the subsequent development of anxiety
over subsequent false alarms forms the core of panic disorder. A diagram
of this model of panic disorder is presented in Figure 2-1.

Based on this model, treatments for panic disorder would involve a
direct attack on learned alarms and anxious apprehension surrounding
the alarms.

The Treatment of Panic

Drug Treatment

Before presenting evidence on nondrug psychological treatments for
panic, it is useful to review very briefly evidence that has accumulated on
the effectiveness of drug treatments. Generally, several classes of drugs
have been studied and/or proposed as possible treatments for panic
disorder: antidepressant medications, including both tricyclic and monoamine oxidase inhibitors (MAOIs); benzodiazepines, including drugs
such as diazepam and alprazolam; beta blockers, best represented by
propranolol; and clonidine, an antihypertensive medication.

ANTIDEPRESSANT MEDICATIONS

Most of the research using antidepressant medications (both tricyclics
and MAOIs) in the treatment of panic attacks has been conducted on
agoraphobics with panic attacks; relatively few studies have focused
directly on panic disorder.

Reviews of this literature reach different conclusions. Ballenger
(1986) and Vittone and Uhde (1985) concluded that pharmacological
treatments generally were effective. On the other hand, Telch, Tearnan,
and Taylor (1983) found reason to question seriously the efficacy of
antidepressant pharmacotherapy for agoraphobia. We now consider
these arguments.

Most of the evidence in support of the efficacy of tricyclics in the
treatment of panic attacks has come from studies using imipramine. A

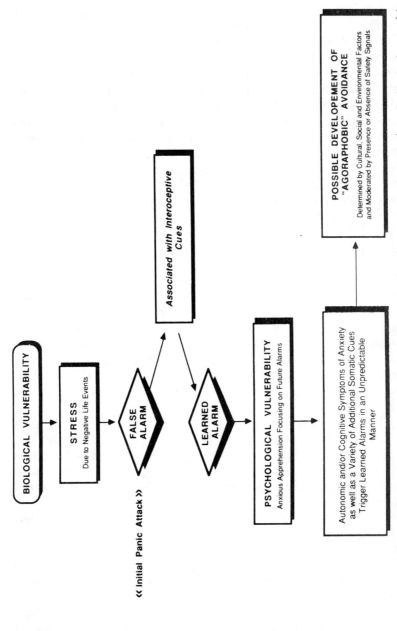

FIGURE 2-1. A model of the etiology of panic disorder. Reprinted with permission from: Barlow, D. H. *Anxiety and its disorders*, 1988. Copyright 1988 by The Guilford Press.

number of uncontrolled clinical trials have generally found imipramine to be effective in the treatment of either panic disorder (Garakani, Zitrin, & Klein, 1984; Munjack *et al.*, 1985; Nurnberg & Coccaro, 1982; Sweeney, Gold, Pottash, & Martin, 1983) or agoraphobia with panic attacks (McNair & Kahn, 1981). Of course, the data from these clinical trials are anecdotal and at best suggestive. But these studies provide a basis for conducting more soundly designed and controlled research.

Eight published double-blind, placebo-controlled studies have reported on the efficacy of imipramine for either agoraphobia with panic attacks or panic disorder. In a series of studies, Klein and his colleagues (Klein, 1964; Klein & Fink, 1962; Zitrin, Klein, & Woerner, 1978, 1980; Zitrin, Klein, Woerner, & Ross, 1983) reported that imipramine was more effective than a placebo, whether given alone or in combination with behavior therapy or supportive therapy, for agoraphobia and for mixed phobics (patients with circumscribed phobias with panic attacks). But they did not find the same effects for simple phobics who typically do not have spontaneous panic attacks. Based on these data, Klein (Klein, 1980; Klein & Rabkin, 1981) has argued that imipramine acts selectively to block panic attacks but has little effect on anticipatory anxiety, which is perhaps best treated with benzodiazepines. These studies have been criticized on methodological grounds (Barlow *et al.*, 1985; Emmelkamp, 1982; Marks, 1981; Mathews *et al.*, 1981) and are challenged further by more recent, well-controlled studies showing that imipramine does have an anti-anxiety effect independent of any antidepressant properties (Kahn *et al.*, 1986). While Klein's argument that imipramine acts specifically on panic attacks may be in jeopardy, these investigations as a whole suggest that imipramine may be helpful in the treatment of panic disorder.

Other controlled studies also have found imipramine useful in treating panic-related problems (Charney & Heninger, 1985; Sheehan, Ballenger, & Jacobson, 1980). In all of the aforementioned studies, imipramine was combined with some other form of therapy, which often included exposure to anxiety-provoking situations or at least encouragement and support for such exposure. The addition of treatment components other than medication leaves open the possibility that the improvement in disorders may have been due to exposure. Indeed, Marks *et al.* (1983) found that when exposure treatment was systematically controlled, imipramine had no significant therapeutic effect despite adequate blood plasma levels. Telch *et al.* (1983) also tested the effects of imipramine alone, imipramine plus intensive *in vivo* exposure, and placebo plus intensive *in vivo* exposure. The results of this study showed that agoraphobics receiving imipramine alone failed to improve on any measures, including measures of panic, but they did show some improvement on measures of depression. The two groups given exposure treatment showed marked improvements on measures of phobic anxiety and avoidance, self-efficacy, panic, and depression. The combined imipramine-exposure group improved significantly more than the placebo–exposure group on measures of phobic anxiety.

The studies by Kahn et al. (1986), Marks et al. (1983), and Telch et al. (1983) clearly call into question the hypothesis that imipramine acts selectively to block panic attacks. In addition, these data raise the possibility that the therapeutic effects of imipramine in treating panic disorders is limited to its facilitative effect on exposure or other psychological treatments. While the apparently well-documented antidepressant and anxiolytic effects of imipramine may be helpful adjuncts for the behavioral treatment of panic disorder, it is not clear that imipramine alone has a selective effect on panic attacks.

Other tricyclic compounds also have been used to treat anxiety disorders. Telch et al. (1983) and Ballenger (1986) have reviewed the literature on clomipramine and suggest that it may be effective in treating agoraphobia with panic attacks as well as obsessive–compulsive disorder. In the largest of these studies (Beaumont, 1977), half of the 480 patients were symptom free at the end of the 12-week trial, and another 20–30% showed significant improvement. However, over 37% of the 765 subjects who started the treatment dropped out of the study, primarily because of the unpleasant side effects of the drug. An open clinical trial (Grunhaus, Gloger, & Birmacher, 1984) also suggested that clomipramine is effective in treating panic.

Other tricyclics, such as desimipramine, nortriptyline, maprotiline, doxepin, and amitriptyline, have been used to treat anxiety problems (Ballenger, 1986). However, there are no published controlled studies that directly compare these tricyclics to each other or to nondrug treatments for panic disorder. Thus, preliminary data suggest that as a class, tricyclic compounds may be generally useful in alleviating some of the symptoms found in panic disorder. But, to date, there are few data supporting the hypothesis that imipramine or any of the other tricyclic compounds specifically blocks panic attacks.

The second class of antidepressant drugs that may be effective in the treatment of agoraphobia and panic disorder are the MAOI. Phenelzine is the MAOI that has been used most often in treating anxiety disorders and apparently the only one for which data from controlled studies are available. Reviews of these data (Ballenger, 1986; Dittrich, Houts, & Lichstein, 1983; Sheehan, 1985; Vittone & Uhde, 1985) generally argue that phenelzine is helpful in improving the symptomatology of agoraphobia and panic disorder. In addition, it appears that phenelzine may be more effective than imipramine, especially for severe cases of agoraphobia and/ or panic disorders. Most of these studies, like imipramine studies, combined the drug treatment with some type of psychotherapy or behavior therapy that most likely encouraged the patients to expose themselves to anxiety-provoking situations. The one published study that compared phenelzine and exposure in a placebo-controlled study with agoraphobics found exposure treatment to be superior to nonexposure treatments and no significant differences between placebo and phenelzine (Solyom, Solyom, LaPierre, Pecknold, & Morton, 1981). Telch et al. (1983) pointed out the similarities between this study and Marks et al.'s (1983) study, which also found imipramine to have little effect independent of exposure treatment. Specifically, antidepressant effects may have been confounded by failure to control adequately for unplanned exposure treatment. In both studies, patients' depression scores were lower than in studies with positive outcomes, suggesting that the antidepressant effects may have contributed to treatment success. That imipramine has been shown to have anxiolytic effects independent of its antidepressant effect (Kahn et al., 1986; Lipman et al., 1986) would seem to argue against this hypothesis.

While a substantial number of studies seem to support the use of antidepressant drugs for the treatment of panic disorder, we agree with Telch et al. (1983) that after considering the methodological flaws in these studies, on the whole the data showing the efficacy of antidepressant medications for the treatment of agoraphobia or panic disorder are not strong at this time. Nevertheless, the weight of the evidence suggests that antidepressants facilitate the effects of exposure treatment but not necessarily by blocking panic directly. Rather, the general anxiolytic effects of these drugs may be the primary contribution to treatment (see Barlow, 1988).

Any therapeutic effect of medication, of course, needs to be weighed against potential negative side effects. Treatment dropout rates are generally recognized as being much higher for antidepressant medications than for nondrug treatments. Given the typical unpleasant side effects associated with these drugs (e.g., dry mouth, sweating, constipation, hypertension), and the need for rather severe dietary restrictions with MAOIs, differences in dropout rate are not unexpected. In addition, even those who most enthusiastically support the use of antidepressant medications for treating panic problems recognize that "relapse . . . after the drug is stopped . . . is much more common than generally believed" (Sheehan, 1985, p. 53). While the research into the causes of relapse after drug treatment have yet to be addressed, it has often been suggested that attributions of control over one's behavior may be a critical factor in determining whether or not a patient relapses.

BENZODIAZEPINES

The second major class of pharmaceutical agents that have been used to treat anxiety problems are the benzodiazepines. These medications have been used most often to treat generalized anxiety and stress rather than disorders associated with panic attacks. Historically, the benzodiazepines have been considered to have little effect in the treatment of panic disorders (Klein, 1980; Sheehan, 1982, 1985). This clinical impression, however, has been challenged by more recent reports showing that some benzodiazepines may be effective in the treatment of panic disorder.

In a double-blind, crossover design, Noyes *et al.* (1984) compared diazepam, a benzodiazepine, and propranolol, a beta blocker. In this study, 20 patients who had either panic disorder or agoraphobia with panic attacks and one patient diagnosed with generalized anxiety disorder were given two trials of each drug, with a 1-week washout period at the beginning of each trial. The median daily dose was 30 mg of diazepam and 240 mg of propranolol hydrochloride. No other formal treatment was provided. Diazepam reduced significantly the number and intensity of panic attacks, while propranolol did not affect panic attacks. Diazepam treatments also reduced significantly phobic symptoms and social impairment, and resulted in scores on several questionnaires and the Hamilton Anxiety Scale. Independent clinical observers rated 86% of the patients as at least moderately improved at the end of the second week of treatment with diazepam, but only 33% of those treated with propranolol were given the same ratings. The authors concluded that benzodiazepines constitute effective short-term treatment for panic-related disorders. In addition, patients who reported predominately somatic symptoms were no more responsive to propranolol than were patients who presented primarily with psychological symptoms.

In a large-scale, multicenter study, Cohn (1981) compared two benzodiazepines—diazepam and alprazolam—with a placebo treatment in a 4-week double-blind study. While the patients used in this large-scale study were described as mixed "anxiety syndrome" rather than given specific anxiety diagnoses, the study is noteworthy because of the large number of subjects treated: 396 patients received diazepam, 407 were treated with alprazolam, and 365 received a placebo. Both diazepam and alprazolam were more effective than the placebo in relieving anxiety symptoms as measured by the patients' and physicians' ratings of improvement and as scored on the Hamilton Anxiety Scale. Alprazolam was significantly more effective than diazepam, suggesting that this newer form of benzodiazepine may be helpful in treating anxiety and perhaps panic.

Alprazolam, marketed as Xanax, is the newest drug in the benzodiazepine family. It is a triazolobenzodiazepine that reaches its peak blood levels 1–2 hours after oral ingestion; its half-life is 12.2 hours (Cohn, 1981). Unlike diazepam, which had been considered ineffective in treating panic disorder, alprazolam has been advanced as a specific treatment for panic disorder. More importantly, several studies have confirmed the usefulness of alprazolam in treating panic attacks.

Chouinard, Annable, Fontaine, and Solyom (1982) completed one of the first controlled studies in which panic patients were treated with alprazolam. Twenty patients with panic disorder and 30 with generalized anxiety disorder were randomly assigned to either alprazolam or a placebo in this double-blind study. All patients received short-term behavior therapy consisting of relaxation training and desensitization four times a week for the last 4 weeks of the treatment program. Two subjects dropped out of the drug group and three dropped out of the placebo group. The results showed that alprazolam was significantly better than placebo in treatment of both disorders, as reflected in improved scores on the Hamilton Anxiety Scale, physicians' ratings, and patients' ratings of anxiety symptoms. While the authors did not report on changes in panic attacks directly, they did find that somatic complaints were most responsive to alprazolam treatment. We have found that behavioral treatment of panic disorder also has its clearest effect on somatic symptoms (Cerny, Sanderson, & Barlow, 1984), which may account for the fact that after 4 weeks of behavioral treatment there was no difference between the placebo and alprazolam groups on any of the dependent variables. Drowsiness, weakness, and fatigue were the most common side effects of alprazolam.

While alprazolam appears to hold some promise as an adjunctive treatment for panic disorder, enthusiasm for this drug is tempered by several reports of iatrogenic effects of alprazolam treatment. Alprazolam treatment of panic has been associated with precipitation of serious hostility (Rosenbaum, Woods, Groves, & Klerman, 1984) and liver impairment (Judd, Norman, Mariott, & Burrows, 1986). In addition, the reports of drug tolerance and dependency with concomitant difficulty in discontinuing alprazolam use have not been infrequent (Klein, Uhde, & Post, 1986; Levy, 1984; Noyes et al., 1984; Vital-Herne, Brenner, & Lesser, 1985). While very carefully planned withdrawal schedules may attenuate somewhat negative withdrawal reactions, the potential for dependency syndromes is clearly present. Also, because the relapse rate for panic attacks is extremely high when alprazolam is stopped (approaching 100%) (DuPont & Pecknold, 1985; Fyer et al., 1987), the best use of alprazolam may be as an adjunctive treatment in cases that are particularly recalcitrant to treatment by behavior therapy alone.

BETA BLOCKERS

Propranolol is the beta blocker that has been most frequently suggested as a possible treatment for panic disorder. Early studies suggested that mitral valve prolapse (MVP) shares with panic disorder some of the same clinical symptoms (Dittrich et al., 1983) and that MVP was more common among patients with panic disorder than among normal controls (Crowe, Pauls, Kerber, & Noyes, 1981). Other studies reported that propranolol, which is used to treat MVP, may also be effective in reducing panic symptoms. Later studies, however, have found no significant difference in MVP incidence among panic patients than among other diagnostic categories (Kane, Woerner, Zeldis, Kramer, & Saravay, 1981) nor is the incidence of panic disorder higher among MVP patients than among control subjects (see Chapter 3). These results certainly call into question the hypothesis that MVP is differentially associated with panic disorder. In addition, several studies have found that propranolol by itself is not as effective as other drugs in reducing anxiety symptoms (Hallstrom, Treasaden, Edwards, & Lader, 1981; Noyes et al., 1984; Tyrer & Lader, 1974). Therefore, propranolol is not usually recommended as the sole treatment for panic attacks. On the other hand, propranolol may help increase the therapeutic effects of other anxiolytic medications. Hallstrom et al. (1981) found that the combination of propranolol and diazepam was more effective than diazepam alone or a placebo in relieving anxiety symptoms. Likewise, Sheki and Patterson (1984) found a synergistic effect when a combination of propranolol and alprazolam was used to treat 16 panic patients in an open clinical trial. Because propranolol is helpful in treating MVP symptoms, these drug combinations may be especially helpful for panic patients who also have MVP. Because neither of the preceding studies commented on the incidence of MVP among their subjects, this treatment possibility is purely speculative.

CLONIDINE

Finally, we want to comment briefly on another type of drug, clonidine, which is an alpha agonist often used to treat hypertension. Clonidine reportedly reduced anxiety symptoms significantly more in depressed patients than in normal controls (Uhde et al., 1981). More to the point, Hoehn-Saric, Merchant, Keyser, and Smith (1981) compared the effects of clonidine and a placebo on 9 generalized anxiety disorder and 14 panic patients in a double-blind crossover design. Clonidine was more effective than the placebo in reducing anxiety levels as measured by the Hamilton Anxiety Scale, physicians' ratings, and patients' ratings. These treatment effects were described as modest because most patients were less anxious but not asymptomatic. The panic and generalized anxiety disorder patients responded similarly to the medication trial. While clonidine is not well supported as a treatment for panic attacks, the fact that it has been found helpful by some panic patients raises the possibility that any drug that has a noticeable calming effect may be a useful adjunctive treatment for panic attacks.

SUMMARY

We have much to learn about drug treatments and underlying neurobiological processes associated with anxiety and panic. Much of what we do know is reviewed elsewhere (e.g., Barlow, 1988). Pending future research, our preliminary conclusions are that both antidepressants and benzodiazepines can be effective adjuncts to exposure-based treatments for agoraphobia. It also seems likely to us that both classes of drugs are primarily anxiolytics rather than panicolytics specifically, although their effects are mediated by rather different neurobiological mechanisms. But large differences in relapse rates seem evident. Relapse after withdrawal from antidepressants appears far less than that associated with benzodiazepines (Barlow, 1988). Initial dropout rates, however, are somewhat higher with antidepressants.

The frontier of research in this area will surround interactions between drug treatment and psychological treatment, particularly newer psychological treatments that directly target panic rather than agoraphobic avoidance behavior.

Psychological Treatment

Since the early 1980s, we may have discovered something unprecedented in the annals of psychotherapy research. Preliminary evidence from a number of centers around the world suggests that we can eliminate panic. Of course, the aforementioned exposure-based treatments for agoraphobia also seem to eliminate panic in some cases. Drugs also may eliminate panic, as long as one remains on the drug in the majority of cases. But with specifically targeted psychological treatments such as described in this book, panic seems to be eliminated in close to 100% of cases, and these results are maintained at follow-up periods of up to 2 years. This may turn out to be one of the more important developments in the history of psychotherapy.

Unfortunately, these conclusions are only tentative. The evidence is based on a clinical series of patients treated without appropriate controls or comparisons. Preliminary evidence from only one controlled study conducted at our center is available and this is reviewed here next.

Based on our model, both reduction of anxious apprehension concerning future false or learned alarms and elimination of escapist action tendencies associated with the alarm are essential for treatment success. These are best accomplished through the reproduction of and exposure to the somatic symptoms of panic. This type of exposure has been administered in a variety of different ways, accompanied by different explanations for its effectiveness. Other explanations are mentioned here subsequently. Nevertheless, all psychological treatments for panic with any demonstrable success have this core ingredient.

Like all new discoveries there are some interesting early examples of this approach, which were either misinterpreted or ignored. In Wolpe's classic early work, CO_2 inhalations were a common but largely overlooked component of his anxiety-reduction procedures. Generally, inhaling CO_2 was conceptualized as facilitating relaxation and, therefore, promoting the reciprocal inhibition of anxiety. In fact, this may have been a very effective procedure for systematically exposing panic-ridden patients to their feared cues in the benign setting of the therapist's office (Wolpe, 1958). In this sense, other early reports can also be reinterpreted. Orwin (1973) treated eight agoraphobics with "the running treatment," wherein patients were instructed to sprint until breathless and then approach or enter a feared situation. Running, of course, produced many of the somatic signs of panic resulting in systematic exposure to these cues. This recalls some of the early panic-provocation work using exercise (e.g., Cohen & White, 1950).

Watson and Marks (1971), in one of the aforementioned studies, reported the then-puzzling finding that imaginal flooding to relevant phobic cues (imagining an intensely vivid scene depicting phobic cues) was no more effective than irrelevant flooding (being eaten by tigers) in a group composed largely of agoraphobics. In fact, irrelevant flooding produced significantly greater therapeutic effects on subjective anxiety! This is understandable if one considers that interoceptive cues produced by irrelevant flooding are the primary phobic cues.

One of the most interesting early reports along these lines was that of Bonn, Harrison, and Rees (1971). Following up on the origins of provoking panic in the laboratory using lactate, Bonn *et al.* carried this procedure to its logical conclusion, from the point of view of treatment, by administering it repeatedly to 33 patients. While panic was not directly measured, this procedure seemed quite successful. Interestingly, this result was totally ignored. In another early series, Haslam (1974) treated 16 subjects, 10 of whom panicked following a sodium lactate challenge with repeated CO_2 inhalation. Nine of the 10 patients who panicked with lactate demonstrated marked improvement after 6 weeks of CO_2 inhalation treatment. Other early case reports or clinical series by Latimer (1977) and Lum (1976) reported on diverse procedures such as CO_2 inhalation or voluntary hyperventilation, which seemed to result in substantial improvement in cases of what we now call panic disorder.

MODELS OF TREATMENT

Generally, three explanations are offered for the success of these clinical trials (e.g., Rapee, 1987). One tradition espoused by Lum (1976) and Ley (1985) attributes panic to the effects of chronic hyperventilation. Treatment then involves breathing retraining, such that hyperventilatory episodes are precluded (e.g., Kraft & Hooguin, 1984).

A second school of thought focuses on the catastrophic misinterpretation or mislabeling of otherwise normal somatic events as the cause of panic. Treatment then involves the correction of these cognitive distortions (e.g., Beck & Emery, 1985). Several investigators have combined these rationales. For example, Clark, Salkovskis, and Chalkley (1985); Salkovskis, Jones, and Clark (1986); and Rapee (1985) used voluntary room-air hyperventilation and subsequent breathing retraining to educate their patients on more proper attributions for their somatic symptoms. These investigators all emphasize cognitive reattribution. But they also suspect, much as do Lum (1976) and Ley (1985), that a vulnerability to hyperventilation exists in these patients as reflected in low resting pCO_2 measures. In a preliminary study recalling the early work of Cohen (e.g., Cohen & White, 1950), Salkovskis and his colleagues (Salkovskis, Jones, & Clark, 1984; Salkovskis et al., 1986) replicated the finding that panic patients presented with low resting pCO_2. But in an interesting twist, they observed that pCO_2 levels rose to within normal range after successful treatment. Future efforts must be directed at replicating this finding and determining whether changes in pCO_2 levels are specifically due to changes in breathing retraining or are simply the result of any successful panic reduction procedure. Similarly, it will be important to determine whether the oft-observed low pCO_2 levels in panic patients imply something specific about the nature of panic or constitute just another one of many biological markers of chronic overarousal associated with anxiety.

Finally, pure exposure to somatic cues occasioned by any number of provocation procedures such as hyperventilation, CO_2 inhalation, lactate infusion, and so on, has been advocated as the important component for treatment for all of the aforementioned reasons. At present, it is difficult to untangle these explanations because all case studies and clinical replication series advocating one or the other of these approaches have typically included all three components. For example, clinicians emphasizing exposure to either CO_2 inhalation sensations or room-air hyperventilation also employ cognitive procedures in which patients are educated about the source of their somatic symptoms (Clark et al., 1985; Griez & van den Hout, 1983, 1986). Typically, current treatment protocols, including the following one, quite purposely include a combination of these procedures (e.g., Barlow, Cohen, et al., 1984). At this early state in the development of psychological treatments for panic, we have not yet begun to dismantle the treatment package in an attempt to identify the essential components. Therefore, we assume for the moment that these treatment approaches are very similar in their operations and that their effectiveness relates to the preceding model of panic.

CONTROLLED STUDIES

Because of the recency of our emerging conceptualization of the psychological treatment of panic, controlled studies are only beginning to appear. In an early study at our center, we treated patients with panic disorder, as well as patients with generalized anxiety disorder, with a broad-based treatment approach, including all of the aforementioned components. When compared to a waiting-list control group, treated patients demonstrated significant improvement on all measures (Barlow, Cohen, et al., 1984). More importantly, these treatment gains were maintained and even strengthened during a follow-up period averaging a year. Several other early studies also suggest an advantage for this approach. For example, Bonn, Readhead, and Timmons (1984) added a respiratory-control training procedure to a standard in vivo exposure treatment for a group of agoraphobics. This approach was compared to the standard in vivo exposure treatment alone. While few differences emerged at posttest, the small group of individuals receiving respiratory control training were significantly better at 6-month follow-up.

In a clinical replication series with a similar goal, we treated 32 patients with panic disorder either with ($N = 16$) or without agoraphobia (Klosko & Barlow, 1987). While this was not a controlled study, both groups of patients received nearly identical treatments with the following exception. The patients with panic disorder without agoraphobia received systematic exposure to interoceptive cues. The patients with agoraphobia, on the other hand, received more standard exposure-based treatments to external situations for the most part. Up-to-date diary measures of panic episodes revealed some interesting differences in terms of reductions in panic between the two groups. Forty percent of the agoraphobics were panic free after treatment, which is consistent with results on the elimination of panic from other studies of exposure-based treatments for agoraphobia. But fully 80% of the patients with panic disorder were free of panic after treatment. These data suggest that directly attacking panic by exposure to and reinterpretation of internal somatic cues may be a crucial factor in treatment.

Finally, Griez and van den Hout (1986), following up their earlier work, carried out a crossover comparison in 14 patients where CO_2 inhalation was compared with a beta blocker, propranolol. Both treatments were administered for the very brief period of 2 weeks and were separated by a 2-week intermission. Perhaps because of this brevity, no significant differences in percentage reduction of panic attacks were apparent. CO_2 inhalations reduced panic by approximately 50%, while propranolol produced a 38% reduction. However, even in this brief 2-week period, systematic CO_2 inhalations almost eliminated the fear of having another panic attack. Reductions in this measure were significant when compared to propranolol. Therefore, it is possible that panic attacks themselves would have been eliminated if treatments were extended a bit in view of the elimination of anxiety about panic, consistent with the preceding model.

THE ALBANY STUDY

We now have preliminary results from one large controlled trial on the psychological treatment of panic that has been going on in our center since 1983, using the treatment protocol presented in this book. This study was restricted to patients suffering from panic disorder without the complication of substantial avoidance behavior. In other words, individuals with agoraphobia were excluded. Thus, the focus was very clearly on assessing and treating panic.

After careful screening via the Anxiety Disorders Interview Schedule, patients were assigned to one of four groups. One group comprised patients assigned to a waiting-list condition to provide appropriate comparisons at posttreatment. Thus, these patients underwent all assessments but received no treatment during a 15-week period. To the basic interoceptive exposure strategy were added either cognitive procedures, based largely on the work of Beck and Emery (1985), or relaxation procedures. A third group received a combination. Cognitive procedures revolved around identifying automatic catastrophic thoughts concerning physical sensations and attributing them to normal bodily processes. Relaxation procedures involved extensive training in individual muscle relaxation and control and generally followed the outline provided by Bernstein and Borkovec (1973).

At this time, we have finished treating over 20 panic patients, while another 15 subjects have completed the waiting-list period. Although the treated patients were distributed across all three treatment groups, most (13) were in the combined treatment condition. A description of this combined treatment protocol forms the heart of this book.

Data on panic frequency taken from our *Weekly Record* panic diary (see Chapter 3) are presented in Figure 2-2. Data were not complete for a few subjects, accounting for the somewhat lower N. Substantial reduction in panic frequency was noted in the treatment group, with fully 82% reporting no panic at posttreatment (see Figure 2-2). Nobody in the treatment group deteriorated. Some reductions in panic frequency were also noted in the waiting-list group, although two patients deteriorated. Of the waiting-list group, 31% reported no panic after treatment.

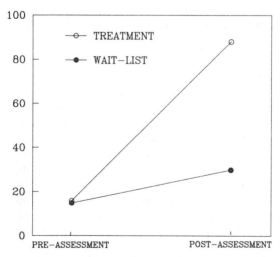

FIGURE 2-2. Percentage of group reporting no panic.

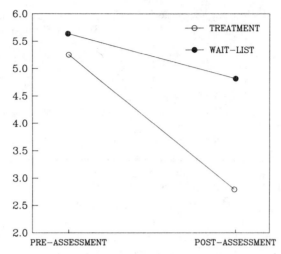

FIGURE 2-3. Clinicians' ratings of severity (on a scale of 0 to 8).

Clinicians' ratings of severity presented in Figure 2-3 also indicate a marked advantage for the treatment group. Follow-up assessments are incomplete, but data recently collected from these patients (Barlow & Craske, 1986), as well as patients from an earlier study (Barlow, Cohen, *et al.*, 1984), indicate a full maintenance of treatment gains. This absence of relapse suggests a fundamental alteration in panic vulnerability although the results are certainly preliminary at this point in time. Until the study is complete, it is not possible to speak of specific contributions made by cognitive or relaxation procedures.

PERCENTAGE OF SUCCESS IN OTHER CENTERS

These are dramatic, if preliminary results. But despite a careful experimental analysis and the resulting confidence with which we can attribute the results to treatment, the information would be of little value if the evidence for treatment effectiveness came only from our center alone. Now we have a series of cases treated in other centers around the world utilizing this general approach that, while uncontrolled, provide equally dramatic evidence on the reduction or elimination of panic.

For example, Gitlan *et al.* (1985) treated 11 patients with panic disorder and reported complete elimination of panic in 10 of these

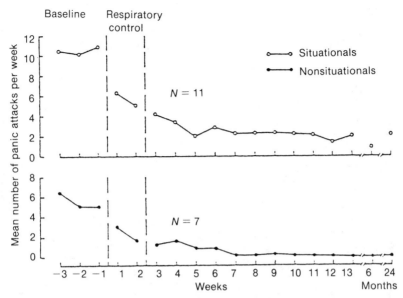

FIGURE 2-4. Effect of respiratory control on panic attacks. Reprinted with permission from: Clark, D. M., Salkovskis, D. M., & Chalkley, A. J. Respiratory control as a treatment for panic attacks. *Journal of Behavior Therapy and Experimental Psychiatry*, 1985, *16*, 23–30. Copyright 1985 by Pergamon Journals, Ltd.

patients at posttreatment. Clark *et al.* (1985) as well as Salkovskis *et al.* (1986) treated panic directly in a number of patients suffering from panic disorders either with or without agoraphobia. These patients were termed "situational" if their panics occurred in primarily agoraphobic situations that they tended to avoid, or "nonsituational" if little or no agoraphobic avoidance was present. The results from Clark *et al.*, presented in Figure 2-4, also indicate nearly total elimination of panic. Finally, a recent series by Beck (1988) seems to confirm and extend the remarkable finding that psychological treatments can eliminate panic. Beck's results with 25 patients are presented in Figure 2-5.

Although uncontrolled, these outcomes from different centers around the world would seem to demonstrate the generality of the findings observed under controlled conditions in our center. Nevertheless, a long road lies ahead if we are to confirm and extend these preliminary findings. Procedural questions revolve around the relative contribution of various components of these sometimes diverse procedures. While all techniques seem to have at their core exposure to

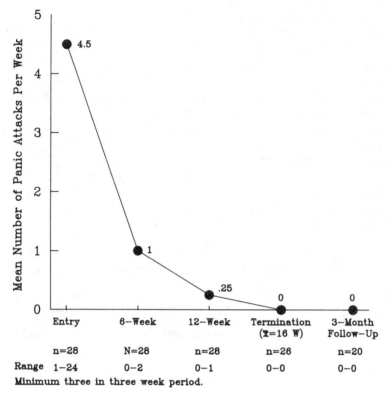

FIGURE 2-5. Number of panic attacks per week over time: Response to treatment. Reprinted with permission from: Beck, A. T. Cognitive approaches to panic disorder: Theory and therapy. In S. Rachman & J. D. Maser (Eds.), *Panic: Psychological perspectives*, 1988. Copyright 1988 by Lawrence Erlbaum Associates.

interoceptive sensations, different emphases are placed on cognitive components and respiratory-control components, as well as on the importance of basic education on the origins of somatic symptoms associated with the nature of panic.

PANIC REDUCTION DURING EXPOSURE TREATMENTS FOR AGORAPHOBIA

One remaining question can now be considered. Why does *in vivo* exposure to external situations have a moderate panic reduction effect in agoraphobics? One possibility is that for those patients with "situational" panics, exposing them to these feared settings has the same effect as inhaling CO_2 or experiencing the effects of sodium lactate infusions. That is, panic attacks are repeatedly provoked under rather benign therapeutic conditions. To the extent that panics or periods of intense anxiety occur, this may be one of the major indicators for successful outcome. For example, Michelson, Mavissakalian, and Marchione (1985) and to a lesser extent Barlow, Cohen, et al. (1984) demonstrated that reduction in anxiety and panic during in vivo exposure were the best predictors of outcome. Furthermore, high autonomic responding, which may reflect an increased tendency to experience anxiety and panic, has been a significant predictor of outcome in many studies (e.g., Vermilyea, Boice, & Barlow, 1984). It is possible, then, that one important procedural contribution of in vivo exposure is the ability of this technique to provoke panic repeatedly. In any case, it seems that we have a successful treatment for panic. A detailed presentation of this protocol constitutes the remainder of this book.

3

Diagnosing and Assessing
Panic Disorder

Organic Conditions Associated with Panic
and Anxiety Symptoms

Before beginning the sometimes difficult process of diagnosing panic disorder, one must screen for a variety of physical problems that produce panic-like symptoms (Hall, 1980; Mackenzie & Popkin, 1983; McCue & McCue, 1984). This does not mean that the presence of one or more of these problems rules out panic disorder. In fact, though panic disorder may exist independently of these disorders, various physical conditions might interact with panic disorder in a way that exacerbates its effects.

Of course, diagnosing these conditions is usually not an issue for mental health professionals because clients most often bring their first panic attack either to emergency rooms or to the office of their primary care physician, where they are screened for these disorders. Only then are they referred to mental health professionals, very often to the surprise of the patient, who assumed that the causes were organic. Nevertheless, determining the presence of these disorders and whether they are being managed properly medically (if management is indicated) is important even if the panic disorder does exist separately. At the very least, the patient should be educated about the relationship among the disorders. In fact, there are numerous physical conditions that may produce these symptoms. For that reason, we present brief descriptions of some of the primary disorders that mimic panic.

Hypoglycemia

Hypoglycemia, which refers to low blood sugar levels, is one of the more common disorders associated with panic. The symptoms of hypoglycemia include sweating, palpitations, weakness, dizziness, faintness, and tremor. Hypoglycemia has various causes—some acute, others more chronic—but clients ordinarily very quickly come to recognize hypoglycemic symptoms and take corrective action to alter blood sugar levels, usually through more frequent intake of foods. One of our clients reported numerous panics, but one would occur quite predictably at approximately 4:00 P.M. every day. In fact, it seemed that the symptoms of hypoglycemia were triggering this particular attack and a small snack prevented it. However, the panic disorder remained and required treatment.

Hyperthyroidism

Hyperthyroidism is a common endocrine disorder that causes restlessness, shortness of breath, palpitations, and tachycardia, as well as tremor and sweating. These symptoms can be very similar to panic. It is also noteworthy that this disorder occurs eight times more frequently in women than in men, with a similar age of onset to panic disorder.

Hypoparathyroidism

This syndrome is characterized by deficiencies in secretions of the parathyroid hormone. The biological results are a depressed concentration of calcium and elevations of phosphate in blood plasma. In extreme cases, panic-like attacks may occur.

Cushing Syndrome

Cushing syndrome, which results from increased circulating levels of cortisol, can sometimes develop during a prolonged period of psychological stress. While acute anxiety and panic are sometimes observed during this disorder, depression is a more common reaction.

Pheochromocytoma

This condition refers to a tumor, generally found in the adrenal glands, that causes excessive secretion of the catecholamines norepinephrine and epinephrine. This disorder very closely mimics panic because the effects of the disorder are to exaggerate the normal secretion of catecholamines that would occur during either stressful periods or preparation for purposeful activity. The symptoms, of course, are identical to those that would occur with any sudden increase in catecholamines as a result of stress or anxiety.

Temporal-Lobe Epilepsy

This form of epilepsy has been associated with a wide range of emotional and sexual disorders including anxiety. Once again, many of the symptoms of panic, such as sweating and palpitations, and even derealization, can result from temporal-lobe epilepsy. To properly diagnose this condition, electroencephalographic (EEG) recordings are required.

Hyperventilation or Caffeine Intoxication

In addition to the aforementioned disorders, a variety of conditions that have been used to provoke panic in the laboratory may be associated with panic attacks and should be ruled out at initial interview. These include acute hyperventilation and excessive intake of caffeine (Barlow, 1988). Hyperventilation is a common response during times of acute stress and seems to be implicated in exacerbating many cases of panic attacks. For this reason, as outlined in our treatment protocol, breathing retraining has a standard place in any psychological treatment of panic. However, many pathways to panic seem independent of hyperventilation (Barlow, 1988). This would seem to rule out the interesting hypothesis that hyperventilation is somehow the cause of panic or even a necessary condition for its occurrence.

The effects of caffeine in provoking panic also may be robust. As Boulenger, Uhde, Wolff, and Post (1984) point out, most people with panic avoid sources of caffeine because they have learned that it exacerbates their panic symptoms. But some have not made this connection. Recently we administered the Anxiety Disorders Interview Schedule (ADIS; described in detail herein later) to a woman who presented with panic disorder after referral from her primary care physician. When asked about coffee-drinking habits or other sources of caffeine intake, she replied that she liked coffee but did not drink to excess. Specification of intake as required on the ADIS, revealed that she prepared and consumed three 10-cup vats of coffee per day! She was referred back to her physician for supervised withdrawal from caffeine addiction before reassessing panic symptomatology. Detailed questions regarding caffeine consumption are included in the ADIS and should be a routine part of any examination of anxiety disorders.

Audiovestibular System Disturbance

In a very interesting pilot study with potentially important implications, Jacob, Moller, Turner, and Wall (1985) administered an otoneurological examination to 21 patients with either panic disorder or agoraphobia with panic attacks who also reported dizziness, fear of falling, or unsteadiness during their panic attacks. The results indicate that up to two-thirds of the patients had abnormal findings on two or more vestibular tests while almost half were found to have a positive audiological test. The authors point out that it is not yet clear whether these findings are specific to patients with panic disorder compared to other psychiatric diagnoses. In addition, even if the findings do turn out to be specific for panic patients, it is very possible that anxiety influences the parameters of vestibular tests. Nevertheless the endogenous sensations of disturbed audiovestibular functioning may be frightening to panic patients even if they do not cause panic disorder.

Mitral Valve Prolapse

The condition that has unquestionably received the greatest attention in relation to possible organic etiologies of panic is mitral valve prolapse. Mitral valve prolapse (MVP) is characterized in its extreme form by chest pain, palpitations, headaches, and giddiness, accompanied by an unusual and difficult to characterize systolic murmur. As noted in Chapter 2, the early excitement concerning the relation of panic disorder to MVP was caused by the fact that a series of early studies reported a high percentage of patients with recurrent panic attacks who also presented with MVP

(Crowe, Pauls, Slymen, & Noyes, 1980; Gorman, Fyer, Gliklich, King, & Klein, 1981; Grunhaus, Gloger, Rein, & Lewis, 1982; Kantor, Zitrin, & Zeldis, 1980; Pariser et al., 1979). These early data excited a flurry of speculation that MVP might be a biological marker for panic in a substantial number of patients. However, more recent and more sophisticated examinations using echocardiogram procedures have failed to confirm the earlier reported high prevalence of MVP. Studies from around the country, notably by Shear, Devereux, Kramer-Fox, Mann, and Frances (1984), as well as Mavissakalian, Salerni, Thompson, and Michelson (1983), found the prevalence of MVP to be no greater than found in the normal population.

Looking at it from a different perspective, Mazza, Martin, Spacavento, Jacobsen, and Gibbs (1986) surveyed the incidence of panic or other anxiety disorders in MVP patients. They found no differences in prevalence of anxiety disorder in MVP patients versus controls without MVP. Hartmann, Kramer, Brown, and Devereux (1982) who found similar results, suggests that the high prevalence of MVP in anxiety disorders was due to biased screening. Finally, Gorman et al., (1981) reported that panic patients with and without MVP responded equally well to imipramine and Crowe et al. (1980) found a similar pattern of inheritance for panic disorder whether MVP was present in the index case or not, suggesting that MVP is not related in any important way to panic. One major problem here is that it is exceedingly difficult to diagnose MVP reliably because even experienced cardiologists often disagree (Dager, Comess, Saal, & Dunner, 1986). When these diagnostic methodological issues are clarified, we may discover that MVP can exacerbate an existing panic disorder. Until that time, a diagnosis of MVP carries with it no implication for treating panic disorder beyond educating the patient on its benign nature.

Summary

There is little question that the aforementioned various physical disorders can produce symptoms that mimic panic. For this reason, it is understandable that various clinicians suggest from time to time that a substantial proportion of panic disorders may be caused by one or another of these physical problems. What is overlooked is that these two conditions may well exist independently, as more recent evidence has suggested is the case with MVP. What is also often overlooked, even in the case of MVP, is that the presence of a physical disorder producing several anxiety-like symptoms may exacerbate an existing panic disorder by contributing to the negative-feedback cycle discussed in Chapter 2 that seems to produce full-blown panic attacks. Whether the organically caused symptoms are endocrinological (as in hyperthyroidism), vestibular, or cardiovascular (as in MVP), a panic patient may have become overly sensitive to certain patterns of internal physical changes. Patients who have developed learned alarms to one or more of these patterns through a process of interoceptive conditioning and misattribution are more likely to spiral into full-blown panic attacks than if the sensations produced by the physical disorder were not present. Similarly, those patients without panic disorder experiencing one or more of these physical problems do not seem to experience the subjective sensations of anxiety or panic. The ultimate test is whether the patient with a physical disorder stops panicking once the disorder is properly diagnosed, treated, and thoroughly explained. If not, then it is probably time to deal with the panic disorder in its own right.

The Classification of Panic Disorder

We have learned much about the nature of panic during the last few years, although there still is a great deal that we do not know. Some of this new information was presented in the first chapter. Revisions to DSM-III have incorporated several major changes in the category of panic disorder based in part on this information. At least two of these changes should have major treatment implications. First, the category of agoraphobia with panic attacks will no longer be part of DSM-III. Rather, this category will be subsumed under panic disorder. Within panic disorder, agoraphobic avoidance behavior will simply be rated as mild, moderate, or severe. There will also be a catagory for panic disorder without agoraphobic avoidance, which is likely to be little used. The following data indicate that out of 100 consecutive panic disorder cases, all presented with at least mild avoidance. Cases without avoidance may exist in other settings, however, such as cardiology clinics (e.g., Mukerji, Beitman, Alpert, Hewett, & Basha, 1987). Panic disorder with moderate or severe agoraphobic avoidance will correspond roughly to the old DSM-III category of agoraphobia with panic attacks. The evidence that agoraphobic avoidance is a subsequent complication of unexpected panic attacks is now very strong (Barlow, 1986).

This reorganization will recognize that avoidance behavior or other means of coping with unexpected panics are on a continuum. Recently, we interviewed 100 consecutive panic disorder patients and catagorized any avoidance behavior that might accompany their panics as either mild, moderate, or severe (Craske, Sanderson, & Barlow, 1987; Sanderson & Barlow, 1986). These are the preliminary data: mild avoidance, 58/100; moderate avoidance, 35/100; severe avoidance, 7/100. Based on this analysis, the majority of patients present with only mild avoidance (but none present with no avoidance). Thus, the major focus of treatment for these individuals should probably be on panic.

A substantial number of individuals also present with moderate avoidance (and in a few cases severe avoidance). We suggest, based on emerging evidence (Barlow, 1988), that treatment for most of these individuals will be incomplete without directly attacking their panic syndrome. Nevertheless, the complication of severe avoidance behavior also requires extensive intervention. Procedures developed in our clinic for targeting avoidance behavior are presented elsewhere (Barlow & Waddell, 1985) and are not addressed directly in this treatment manual.

A second major revision to panic disorder is found in the definition itself. In this definition (presented in Table 3-1), it is noted for the first time that a defining characteristic of the disorder is a pronounced fear of having another attack: "Either four attacks, as defined in criterion A, occurred within a four-week period, or one or more attacks were followed by a period of at least a month of persistent fear of having another attack." This revision emphasizes, in our view, the crucial aspect of panic disorder. Thus, while it is still possible to receive a diagnosis of panic disorder with four unexpected panic attacks in a 4-week period without any fear of having another attack; in all likelihood, this would be a very infrequent occurrence. We suggested in the previous chapter that anxiety over having another panic attack is what differentiates nonclinical panickers from those individuals suffering to the extent that they seek out mental health professionals. The complete criteria for the revised definition of panic disorder are presented in Table 3-1.

The revised definition continues to include a category of agoraphobia without a history of panic disorder. At present this is a bit of a puzzle to clinical investigators because these individuals seldom, if ever, present to clinics for help. However, epidemiologists report that these people do exist in community samples (Weissman & Merikangas, 1985). The resolution of this discrepancy awaits further investigation.

Assessment: General Strategies

With these considerations in mind, it is possible to begin the process of assessing panic disorder. Initial classification as determined during the interview should always be followed by an elaboration of the characteristic and idiosyncratic responses with which the client presents. This process is often called behavioral analysis or behavioral assessment, although it is routine in most clinical situations. While classification will give the clinician some very good clues on which problematic behaviors to assess, the behavioral analysis is the actual process of assessing each client individually to determine the manner in which the disorder presents itself.

For example, two people who are panicking might present with a very different picture depending on their age, social support system, sex, and economic status, as well as the presence or absence of other associated problems. Number and types of panic attacks and their antecedents as well as particular patterns of avoidance behavior or other coping responses also require additional individual assessment. To assume that every client stereotypically fits the criteria as described in the broad and general classification schema, and that no further information is necessary before beginning treatment, would be naive. Detailed steps involved in this process are outlined in recent books (Barlow, 1981; Nelson & Barlow, 1981). Thus, an initial classification of panic disorder will point the clinician in the proper directions for additional assessment.

For our purposes, behavioral assessment simply means that each client's behavior is carefully observed, measured, and analyzed. More importantly, relationships between these problematic behaviors and environmental or organismic variables that may be maintaining them are continually sought. This is really something that most clinicians do routinely; it is just that behavioral assessment and analysis formalizes the activity and ensures a continuing close interaction between the processes of assessment and treatment until the case is terminated.

Another crucial step in assessment is a comprehensive approach to measuring all presenting problems in what has been termed the three major response systems: behavioral or motoric, cognitive or subjective, and physiological or somatic (Barlow, 1981; Lang, 1968, 1977). In panic disorder, the application is particularly clear. Within the behavioral response system one must carefully assess avoidance or other behavioral attempts at coping with panic. Subjective or cognitive aspects requiring assessment include reports of subjective disturbance or intensity of the various symptoms and the hypothesized final consequences of panic (dying, losing control, etc., described more fully in "Clinical Interview"). Physiological or somatic assessment most often involves monitoring autonomic nervous system reactivity accompanying anxiety and panic, such as increased heart rate, respiration, and other physiological signs of arousal.

A goal of assessment, then, is to examine all three of these components of panic disorder as they relate to each other and as they relate to particular features of each individual's environment resulting in an indi-

TABLE 3-1. DSM-III-R Definition of Panic Disorder

A. At some time during the disturbance, one or more panic attacks (discrete periods of intense discomfort or fear) have occurred that were (1) unexpected; i.e., did not occur immediately before or on exposure to a situation that almost always caused anxiety, and (2) not triggered by situations in which the individual was the focus of others' attention.

B. Either four attacks, as defined in criterion A, occurred within a four-week period, or one or more attacks were followed by a period of at least a month of persistent fear of having another attack.

C. At least four of the following symptoms developed during at least one of the attacks:
   (1) shortness of breath (dyspnea) or smothering sensations
   (2) dizziness, unsteady feelings, or faintness
   (3) palpitations or accelerated heart rate (tachycardia)
   (4) trembling or shaking
   (5) sweating
   (6) choking
   (7) nausea or abdominal distress
   (8) depersonalization or derealization
   (9) numbness or tingling sensations (paresthesias)
   (10) flushes (hot flashes) or chills
   (11) chest pain or discomfort
   (12) fear of dying
   (13) fear of going crazy or of doing something uncontrolled

Note: Attacks involving four or more symptoms are panic attacks; attacks involving fewer than four symptoms are limited symptom attacks (see Agoraphobia without History of Panic Disorder).

D. During at least some of the attacks at least four of the C symptoms developed suddenly and increased in intensity within ten minutes of the beginning of the first C symptom noticed in the attack.

E. It cannot be established that an organic factor initiated and maintained the disturbance, e.g., Amphetamine or Caffeine Intoxication, hyperthyroidism.

Note: Mitral valve prolapse may be an associated condition but does not rule out a diagnosis of Panic Disorder.

Subtypes of Panic Disorder

300.21 with agoraphobia

A. Meets the criteria for Panic Disorder.

B. Agoraphobia: Fear of being in places or situations from which escape might be difficult (or embarrassing) or in which help might not be available in the event of a panic attack. (Include cases in which persistent avoidance behavior originated during an actve phase of Panic Disorder, even if the person does not attribute the avoidance behavior to fear of having a panic attack.) As a result of this fear, the person either restricts travel or needs a companion when away from home, or else endures agoraphobic situations despite intense anxiety. Common agorpahobic situations include being outside the home alone, being in a crowd or standing in a line, being on a bridge, and traveling in a bus, train, or car.

TABLE 3-1. (continued)

Specify current severity of agoraphobic avoidance:

Mild: Some avoidance (or endurance with distress), but relatively normal life-style, e.g., travels unaccompanied when necessary, such as to work or to shop; otherwise avoids traveling alone.

Moderate: Avoidance results in constricted life-style, e.g., the person is able to leave the house alone, but not to go more than a few miles unaccompanied.

Severe: Avoidance results in being nearly or completely housebound or unable to leave the house unaccompanied.

In Partial Remission: No current agoraphobic avoidance, but some agoraphobic avoidance during past six months.

In Full Remission: No current agoraphobic avoidance and none during the past six months.

Specify current severity of panic attacks:

Mild: during the past month, either all attacks have been limited symptom attacks (i.e., fewer than four symptoms), or there has been no more than one panic attack.

Moderate: During the past month attacks have been intermediate between "mild" and "severe."

Severe: during the past month, there have been at least eight panic attacks.

In Partial Remission: The condition has been intermediate between "In Full Remission" and "Mild."

In Full Remission: During the past six months, there have been no panic or limited symptom attacks.

300.01 without agoraphobia

A. Meets the criteria for Panic Disorder.
B. Absence of Agoraphobia, as defined above.

Specify current severity of panic attacks, as defined above.

300.22 Agoraphobia without History of Panic Disorder

A. Agoraphobia: Fear of being in places or situations from which escape might be difficult (or embarrassing) or in which help might not be available in the event of suddenly developing a symptom(s) that could be incapacitating or extremely embarrassing. Examples include: dizziness or falling, depersonalization or derealization, loss of bladder or bowel control, vomiting, or cardiac distress. As a result of this fear, the person either restricts travel or needs a companion when away from home, or else endures agoraphobic situations despite intense anxiety. Common agoraphobic situations include being outside the home alone, being in a crowd or standing in a line, being on a bridge, and traveling in a bus, train, or car.
B. Has never met the criteria for Panic Disorder.

Specify with or without limited symptom attacks.

Note. Reprinted with permission from the *Diagnostic and Statistical Manual of Mental Disorders, Third Edition, Revised.* Copyright 1987 American Psychiatric Association.

vidualized idiosyncratic pattern for each client. For example, an elderly woman living in a nursing home obviously would have problems different from those of a male with a large family who finds it difficult to talk about his symptoms. With these considerations in mind, it is possible to outline the actual steps involved in diagnosis and assessment, beginning with the specifics of the clinical interview.

Clinical Interview

We have already mentioned the existence of the ADIS. The ADIS is a structured interview developed over several years for diagnosing anxiety disorders and related problems such as affective disorders. It is capable of ruling out a wide variety of additional disorders. The reliability of this instrument is very high (Barlow, in press). The most recent revision (ADIS-R) is designed for DSM-III-R categories. This instrument is available upon request from our center. Administration of this full schedule would not be called for in every clinical setting, particularly in those settings where clinicians are seeing patients with a variety of disorders. Nevertheless, we recommend some of the specific questions from this structured interview that pertain to panic disorder as outlined herein.

Naturally, some special considerations apply when interviewing clients who may have panic disorder, with or without agoraphobic avoidance, as opposed to other disorders. Panic disorder clients are often terrified of the first interview. For those clients who have difficulty leaving their house in order to come to a clinic or office setting, they will anticipate this visit for hours, days, or even weeks in advance. We have had clients turn around and return home after coming within sight of the clinic door. Most often, these persons are accompanied by a spouse or friend, and this alone will require some special logistical considerations. Occasionally, we make a home visit for the first interview, but we avoid this if at all possible because we are already at a considerable advantage if the client learns that he/she can make it to the clinic.

Therapy often begins during the first 10 minutes of this initial interview, when some clients report experiencing a "full-blown" panic. Naturally, the experienced clinician interrupts the proceedings only briefly to say that he/she is well aware of how the patient is feeling before continuing with specific questions. The strategy here is to make every attempt to get the client to focus on the material at hand. While it may appear that the clinician is simply proceeding with the interview, the secondary purpose of diverting the client's attention from symptoms of panic to specific questions is its therapeutic effect.

In terms of the structure of the initial interview, we recommend the graduated funnel approach (Nelson & Barlow, 1981) for obtaining information. This approach initially involves asking relatively global questions about many areas of the individual's life, including such topics as presenting complaints, existence of other problems, history, and functioning in major areas such as family, marital relationships, and so on. Following the initial broad inquiry, the interviewer gradually focuses on and asks more detailed questions about issues and problems that have been identified as requiring further information. As any clinician knows, it is not at all uncommon to discover that the client's initial complaints are not his/her primary concern, but that more serious problems exist in other areas of functioning. In the special case of panic disorder, clients occasionally will present with complaints of panic and, perhaps, extensive avoidance when, in fact, a severe obsessional process, a psychotic process, or perhaps even unrelated substance abuse is more prominent.

To assess for panic disorder, we use the sequence of questions from the April 1987 version of the ADIS-R (Di Nardo et al., 1985) shown in Table 3-2. A demonstration of the actual process of this interview carried out by Peter A. Di Nardo, who had primary responsibility for constructing the ADIS-R, is presented in the audiotape accompanying the manual.

The first series of questions assesses for the existence of panic with the potential of establishing a diagnosis of panic disorder. Particularly important is the determination of whether an unexpected or uncued panic was implicated in the initiation of the disorder. Only if the occurrence of an unexpected uncued panic is identified does the interviewer continue examining for panic disorder. If panic was always expected ("I thought I'd probably panic when I saw that spider") or cued ("I always get anxious when speaking in front of groups, although I've never had this bad a reaction"), the interviewer skips this portion of the ADIS-R and proceeds to examine panic in the context of other anxiety disorders such as social or simple phobia. If unexpected or uncued panic is established by questions in Table 3-2, these questions are followed by questions on the degree and extent of avoidance behavior or other responses that may have developed for the purpose of coping with unexpected panic.

Variability across time in the pattern of panic and avoidance behavior is also examined directly in the interview. Almost all panic clients report that they experience good days on which they are more active with less avoidance as well as bad days when they may end up totally housebound. Similarly, clients with uncomplicated panic disorder (with little avoidance) may simply panic more frequently. Many female clients report that they are at their worst immediately before or during menstrua-

TABLE 3-2. Panic Disorder Section of the ADIS-R

1. a. (Have you had times when you have felt a sudden rush of intense fear or anxiety or feeling of impending doom?)

    Yes _____ No _____

    If Yes, or uncertain, continue inquiry. Otherwise, skip to Generalized Anxiety Disorder.

2. a. (In what situation(s) have you had these feelings?)

    _____

   b. (Have you had these feelings come "from out of the blue," or while you are at home alone, or in situations where you did not expect them to occur?)

      Yes _____ No _____

      If patient indicates that panic symptoms occur only in a specific situation (public speaking, heights, driving, etc.), further inquiry is necessary to determine if symptoms occur immediately upon exposure to the situation.

   c. (When you are faced with [phobic situation], does the anxiety come on as soon as you enter it, or is it sometimes delayed, or unexpected?)

      Delayed? Yes _____ No _____

      If Yes to 2b or 2c, or if there is any uncertainty about the existence of panic symptoms, continue inquiry. Otherwise, skip to Generalized Anxiety Disorder.

3. (How long does it usually take for the rush of anxiety to peak?)

    _____ minutes

4. (How long does the anxiety usually last at its peak level?)

    _____ minutes

SYMPTOM RATINGS

In this section rate symptoms *only* for anxiety attacks that occur *unpredictably*, in a variety of situations. Anxiety symptoms that are limited to a single stimulus (enclosed places or heights, social situations, obsessional content, etc.) should be rated in the appropriate section.

In some mixed cases, ratings might be completed in both this section and a later section.

A. Rate the severity of each symptom which is *typical* of the most recent attacks, and during the period of most severe attacks. If a symptom is experienced during only some attacks (i.e., it does *not* typically occur during an attack), enclose the rating in parentheses.

   DSM-III-R requires at least one attack in which four symptoms were present. If typical attacks do not include four symptoms, determine if *any* attack has included four symptoms.

B. If the most recent attacks are also the worst attacks, indicate this and enter severity ratings under the "Most recent" column only.

C. Use the following inquiry when rating symptoms:

1. (During the most recent period of attacks, did you experience _____? How severe was it?) If there is any doubt about whether the symptom is typical, ask: (Do you experience this nearly every time you have an attack?)

TABLE 3-2. (continued)

2. (When the attacks were the most severe, did you experience _____?)

D. If the patient reports four or more symptoms per typical panic attack, the interviewer should ask if the patient had attacks in which only one or two symptoms have been present (Question 6). If the patient answers "Yes," the interviewer should go back and rate the severity of those symptoms under the column labeled "Limited symptom attack."

3. (When were the attacks the most severe?)
   From _____ To _____

   a. (How frequent were the attacks during this period?)

   _____

   b. (What made the attacks the most severe you have had?)

   _____

4. (When was your most recent attack?)

   _____

5. Rate the severity of typical symptoms for each period on the following scale:

   Note: Symptoms that are occasionally experienced, but are not typical, should be rated parenthetically.

0	1	2	3	4
|	|	|	|	|
None	Mild	Moderate	Severe	Very severe

   (Did/do you *usually* experience _____ during the attacks?)

	Most recent	Most severe	Limited symptom attack
1. Shortness of breath (dyspnea) or smothering sensations	___	___	___
2. Choking	___	___	___
3. Palpitations or accelerated heart rate (tachycardia)	___	___	___
4. Chest pain or discomfort	___	___	___
5. Sweating	___	___	___
6. Dizziness, unsteady feelings or faintness	___	___	___
7. Nausea or abdominal distress	___	___	___
8. Depersonalization or derealization	___	___	___
9. Numbness or tingling sensations, paresthesias	___	___	___
10. Flushes (hot flashes) or chills	___	___	___
11. Trembling or shaking	___	___	___

TABLE 3-2. (continued)

12. Fear of dying   _____ _____ _____

13. Fear of going crazy or doing something uncon-
    trolled
                                                         _____ _____ _____

If patient reports four or more symptoms per *typical* attack, ask:

6. (Do you have periods [attacks, spells] when you have only one or two of these
   symptoms?)
   Yes _____   No _____

If Yes, go back and rate severity of symptoms under "Limited symptom attack" column.

Note: Diagnosis of Panic Disorder requires presence of four symptoms during at
least one attack. If typical attacks do not include four symptoms, determine if *any*
attack has included four symptoms.

7. a. (During the time that the attacks were most frequent, how often did they occur?)
      _____ per week for _____ weeks

   b. (When was this period?)
      From _____ To _____

      If patient reports full panic attacks (four or more symptoms) and limited attacks,
      obtain frequencies for both types in c and d

   c. (During the past month, how many panics have you had?)
      _____ per week for _____ weeks

   d. (How many attacks have you had in the last 6 months?)
      _____ per month for _____ months

   e. (Since your first attack, has there been a period of time when you were afraid that
      you might have more attacks?)
      Yes _____   No _____

      (When was this?)
      From _____ To _____

   f. (In the last month, how much have you been worrying, or how fearful have you
      been about having another attack?)

0	1	2	3	4	5	6	7	8
No worry/ no fear		Rarely worried/ mild fear		Occasionally worried/ moderate fear		Frequently worried/ severe fear		Constantly worried/ extreme fear

8. (Have there been times when you awake from sleep in a panic?)
   Yes _____   No _____

   If Yes, (When did this occur?)
   From _____ To _____

TABLE 3-2. (continued)

(How often?)

_____ per night

_____ nights per week

9. a. (Do you have any specific thoughts before an attack?)

   b. (Do you have any specific thoughts during an attack?)

10. HISTORY

   (Tell me about your first panic:)

   a. (When did it happen?)

      Month _____ Year _____

   b. (Where were you?)

   c. (Whom were you with?)

   d. (How did it start?)

   e. (What did you do?)

   f. (Were you under any type of stress?)

      Yes _____ No _____

      (What was happening in your life at the time?)

      Specify _____

      (Were you taking any type of drug?) Include alcohol, caffeine.

      Yes _____ No _____

      Type _____ Dose/Amount _____

      (Did you have any physical condition such as inner ear problems, hyperthyroid-
      ism, mitral valve prolapse, pregnancy, hypoglycemia, temporomandibular joint
      dysfunction?)

      Yes _____ No _____

      Specify _____

   g. (Do you remember having similar feelings (maybe milder) any time before this?)

      Yes _____ No _____

      If yes, (When?)

      Month _____ Year _____

      (What was the feeling?)

11. (Have you had periods when the panics became less intense or less frequent?)

    Yes _____ No _____

    If Yes, continue. If No, go to Question 12.

TABLE 3-2. (continued)

(When?) (From __ To __) (Month and year)	(What was going on in your life? How did you get over it? i.e., Did stressor let up or did person develop coping strategy?)	(How did they come back? Changes in life circumstances? Stressor related?)

12. (How do you handle the panics now?)

13. DISTRESS/INTERFERENCE
(How much have the panics interfered with your life, job, traveling, activities, etc.?)

Rate interference on 0–4 scale _____

0	1	2	3	4
None	Mild	Moderate	Severe	Very severe/ grossly disabling

Note. Reprinted with permission from: Di Nardo, P. A., Barlow, D. H., Cerny, J. A., Vermilyea, B. B., Vermilyea, J. A., Himadi, W. G., & Waddell, M. T. Anxiety Disorders Interview Schedule—Revised (ADIS-R), 1985. Copyright 1985 by Phobia and Anxiety Disorders Clinic, State University of New York at Albany.

tion, which seems to provide yet another pattern of heightened physiological sensations capable of spiraling into panic.

One problem that is quite variable across panic disorder is depersonalization or derealization (feelings of unreality on the ADIS-R). In our experience, only a minority of panickers report this problem, but when they do, it is usually reported as the prominent feature of panic and often requires some special therapeutic attention.

Finally, every clinician should examine patterns of cognitions associated with panic and avoidance behavior. Initial questions on this topic are specified on the ADIS-R. Several issues frequently arise in this context. Despite the increasing publicity given to panic and agoraphobia in popular magazines and newspapers, many clients have avoided seeking out health professionals thinking that they are the only persons in the world with such symptoms. They are concerned that the diagnostic process will mean quick institutionalization in the nearest state hospital.

Once relieved of this concern, thoughts of impending catastrophic consequencs associated with anxiety and panic most often fall into one or two categories. First, some agoraphobics will report that if they fall prey to their panic while away from their safe place or person, they will eventually lose control and "go crazy" or "go insane." Second, others report that the ultimate catastrophic consequence is a severe physical problem, usually a "heart attack" followed by death. As noted in Chapter 1, these catastrophic consequences have been separated for more accurate specification on the DSM-III-R symptoms list.

As mentioned, the most important part of the assessment is a determination of the functional relationship between avoidance behavior, cognitive patterns, and panic on the one hand, and associated internal or external cues on the other hand. This is the functional analysis in which maladaptive behaviors and feelings are related to specific events, resulting in individual and idiosyncratic patterns of responses. For example, in one client, health concerns such as apprehension over heart attacks and increases in avoidance behavior might be tightly tied to expected panic attacks. In another client, health concerns and avoidance behavior may be more independent of expected panic resulting in a more functionally autonomous pattern of responses. It is this determination, over and above the initial classification, that is necessary so that the clinician can tailor individually a standardized set of therapy principles to the client.

THE ASSESSMENT OF SAFETY SIGNALS

Once the interviewer establishes the strong possibility of panic disorder, several other areas should be covered during the initial interview. While exploring specific patterns and severity of avoidance behavior even if this behavior does not reach agoraphobic proportions, one should be particularly concerned about the degree of reliance on safety signals such as a safe place, a safe person, or inanimate objects such as unused or empty pill bottles (Rachman, 1984). The interviewer should be sure to clarify the identity of persons who are considered safe. Most often the safe person is a spouse, but occasionally it is another family member or a friend. A safe person, of course, means that the agoraphobic feels comfortable with this person to a degree not achievable either alone or with other people not considered safe. This situation may exist whether or not the client's mobility depends on the safe person. That is, even if no avoidance whatsoever is present, the client may feel differentially safe with some people, and this should be noted. Usually, a person is considered safe because he/she knows about the panics. Even if the safe person does not approve, as is the case with some spouses, clients feel that this person would take them to the hospital or be able to help in some way if incapacitated by panic. Often the safety signal is an animal or inanimate object. While pill bottles are common, sheets of paper with coping statements or other talismans often pick up these qualities.

Once the range of safety signals is determined by interview, it is assumed that these will remain relatively constant because they often represent habits of long standing. Therefore, they are not assessed on a repeated basis, although attention to safety signals becomes an integral part of the treatment program as patients are gradually weaned from these ritualistic props. Naturally, particular attention is paid to a safe person such as a spouse, another family member, or a close friend. But one must also be careful to continue to monitor the use of inanimate objects, such as empty bottles of pills, as well as to determine that no new safety signals are picked up along the way. One relatively common problem is that sheets of paper containing coping statements or other new cognitive strategies become substitutes for empty bottles of pills and pick up ritualistic overtones in their own right. By the end of treatment, clinicians must ensure that these have become fully incorporated into the client's day-to-day functioning such that forgetting a sheet of paper with cognitive strategies written on it will not of itself provoke a panic attack.

Questionnaires

Unfortunately, assessing panic as well as the complication of avoidance behavior and the idiosyncratic safety signals that a client may employ is not a straightforward task. From the point of view of convenience, the ideal procedure would involve asking clients periodically how much they are panicking and how much they are avoiding. A more structured way of accomplishing this is to administer psychometrically sound question- naires periodically that do the asking for the clinician. Questionnaires also have the virtue of well-worked-out phrasing of questions that is consistent from time to time. Structured questionnaires also have the advantage of allowing the clinician to compare his/her client's responses to some well-established norm for persons with similar problems. Unfor- tunately, both periodic informal questions and structured questionnaires require that the desired information be filtered through the client's view of how things seem to be going at that moment. For example, asking a client how many times he/she has panicked in the past week requires, first, that the client remembers each and every panic. This is a task that research on assessment had demonstrated time and again to be very, very difficult, even for the best-intentioned client (Barlow, Hayes, & Nelson, 1984). In addition, the client must remain immune to the ever-present demands inherent in this type of situation—the most common of which is a desire to please the therapist by reporting things are somewhat better than they actually are.

This situation is illustrated from one of our agoraphobics treated several years ago in our clinic. This client, a male in his 40s, presented with a particularly severe case of agoraphobic avoidance associated with panic disorder. He was panicking at a high frequency, and the avoidance behavior was beginning to keep him from his job in a local factory. Progress during treatment always was assessed by asking the client how he was doing. But progress was also assessed by the administration of questionnaires from time to time, as well as periodic direct behavioral observations of avoidance in the client's home situation. The client demonstrated substantial improvement on self-report measures during treatment. This progress was maintained during a 1-year follow-up on these measures. However, periodic direct behavioral observations reflected that most of the initial gains during treatment were largely lost at follow-up.

Despite these caveats, a number of very useful questionnaires with demonstrated reliability and validity now exist. The difficulty is that most of them were devised for panic disorder patients presenting with substantial agoraphobic avoidance. Thus, the emphasis has been on avoidance behavior. Nevertheless, we have found two questionnaires useful. One, the Fear Questionnaire, is widely used; it is brief and has been standardized around the world. The second is actually a pair of questionnaires, the Agoraphobia Cognitions Questionnaire and the Body Sensations Questionnaire. Despite the presence of the term agoraphobia in one of the titles, these are directed at panic and apprehension surrounding panic.

FEAR QUESTIONNAIRE

This widely used measure, developed by Marks and Mathews (1979), appears to possess adequate psychometric properties and yields four main scores: main phobia rating, total phobia rating, anxiety–depression rating, and a global measure of phobic symptoms. In addition, three particularly useful subscores (agoraphobia, blood–injury phobia, and social phobia) are derived (Marks, 1981). This measure requires only a brief administration time, and the agoraphobia subscale, because of its wide acceptance, allows comparison of the severity of agoraphobia to published standards. For example, Mavissakalian (1986) provided data on the validity of the scale and suggested that a cutoff point of 30 on the agoraphobia subscale would identify serious agoraphobia.

AGORAPHOBIA COGNITIONS QUESTIONNAIRE AND BODY SENSATIONS QUESTIONNAIRE

These two companion questionnaires, developed by Chambless, Caputo, Bright, and Gallagher (1984), are designed to assess the cognitive and physiological aspects of panic and anxious apprehension concerning panic, which makes them unique and particularly useful to assess progress during the treatment of panic disorder, either uncomplicated or with extensive avoidance. Both questionnaires possess sound psychometric properties.

Assessing Cognitions

Despite the utility of these and other questionnaires, a word of caution must be offered regarding the assessment of cognitions associated with panic or anxiety. A number of reports have implicated catastrophic or negative thoughts in the maintenance of pathological anxiety (Beck, Laude, & Bohnert, 1974; Last & Blanchard, 1982; May, 1977a, 1977b; Wade, Malloy, & Proctor, 1977). Furthermore, when these negative or catastrophic cognitions are assessed on a pre–post basis, it seems that a number of treatments for panic disorder and agoraphobia result in the amelioration of these thoughts. Of course, as alluded to earlier, cognitive procedures in and of themselves do not seem particularly successful in the treatment of clinical phobias (Biran, Augusto, & Wilson, 1981; Biran & Wilson, 1981; Emmelkamp, 1982; Emmelkamp, Brilman, Kuiper, & Mersch, 1986; Williams & Rappoport, 1983). But the modification of panic-related cognitions may yet prove to be an important index of progress whatever the treatment.

In any case, the assessment of catastrophic thoughts proves to be a very slippery task because these cognitions are extremely variable from time to time and do not seem to covary reliably with treatment effectiveness. In an attempt to look very closely at the pattern of phobic cognitions across time, Last et al. (1984) repeatedly assessed cognitions in agoraphobics under two conditions. During an *in vivo* cognitive assessment, cognitions were directly recorded on a microcassette recorder as subjects freely verbalized any thoughts during exposure sessions at a local shopping mall. In addition, immediately following each *in vivo* assessment occasion throughout treatment, subjects recorded thoughts they recalled having during the exposure period in written form using a thought-lising procedure (Cacioppo & Petty, 1981). All cognitions were classified using a previously developed categorization system including both negative, positive, and neutral thoughts into which thought content could be categorized reliably by raters.

The results of this investigation revealed decreases in negative and catastrophic thoughts from the beginning to the end of therapy, whether cognitive therapeutic procedures were included with the exposure based treatment or not. However, the changes in catastrophic thinking were not related directly to therapeutic success. Many of the changes occurred during baseline when no treatment was in effect. At other times during treatment, cognitions would show marked fluctuations that seemed to bear no relation to progress. It is entirely possible that any changes occurring during infrequent assessment, such as before and after treatment, may simply be an artifact of the timing of the assessment.

For this reason, it seems that the major emphasis of assessment is best placed on panic as well as maladaptive coping procedures such as avoidance behavior, rather than on cognitions per se.

Self-Monitoring Measures

Years of research in behavioral assessment (e.g., Barlow, 1981) has demonstrated that continuous monitoring of behavioral and emotional events is far preferable to periodic recall of these events in terms of accuracy and reliability. These procedures have now been fully incorporated into the assessment and treatment of panic with or without agoraphobic avoidance. Before describing typical self-monitoring procedures for panic and avoidance behavior, it is only fair to warn the clinician that there are a number of drawbacks to self-monitoring. Particularly problematic is the issue of compliance with recording because this does require a certain amount of effort on the part of the client. Procedures have been developed to enhance recording compliance in order to increase the reliability of the obtained data (cf. Barlow, Hayes, & Nelson, 1984).

There are several ways in which we deal with problems of compliance. First, we emphasize the importance of the daily record when we first start seeing the patient. Second, we have at least 1 and sometimes 2 weeks of training and practice with the form during assessment before treatment begins. This can be accomplished conveniently during the initial assessment sessions. Third, we examine systematically the records as they are handed in, particularly in the first few weeks, and we provide detailed corrective feedback on the accuracy and completeness of the record at the time of the session, highlighting in a very positive way compliance with the recordkeeping activity.

Despite the effort involved in this, both on the part of the client and the therapist, the importance of this type of monitoring has emerged clinically time and time again. Accurate record keeping by the client at or near the time of the event has often provided important information that may seem routine to the client and/or spouse and family and, therefore, is not reported at weekly sessions. Particular strategies and thrusts within therapy will often turn on this information.

In treating panic disorder, we employ one self-monitoring form for assessing both panic and generalized anxiety on a day-to-day basis. These forms have been worked out after years of trial and error in our clinic to provide us with the type of information that we find most useful, as well as to make it as easy and convenient for the patient as possible. The number of details required on the forms might be in excess of what the average clinician would need, but all of the information has proved useful at one time or another.

The *Weekly Record* allows one to assess both the background or generalized anxiety and the frequency, intensity, duration, and number of symptoms comprising a panic attack, as well as instances of elevated generalized anxiety that would not meet the criteria for panic attacks. Perceived antecedents or cues associated with these intense anxiety episodes, as well as panic attacks, are also recorded. To indicate levels of generalized anxiety, clients are instructed to record their current anxiety level on a scale of 0 to 8 four times daily. For monitoring intense anxiety and panic, they are asked to record every discrete instance of anxiety that reaches a level of 4 (moderately severe) or higher. For each recording of elevated anxiety or panic, the client includes time of onset and offset of the episode, maximum intensity, anxiety level at offset, and whether it was a panic attack or not (clarified herein later).

A distinction is also made between expected and unexpected panic. Thus, an unexpected panic is defined as the sudden onset of intense fear that occurs unexpectedly, whether there is a clear cue or not. Information about probable antecedents or precipitants to these intense anxiety reactions or panics are obtained in two places. The client is required to record both a brief description of the situation in which the reaction occurs and any thoughts that occur just prior to or during the reaction. The client also provides a brief note regarding the perceived cause of this particular episode and whether it was expected or not. An example of this form as it was filled out by one of our clients is presented in Appendix A. An updated version of this form, along with the instructions that accompany it, may be found in Appendix B. We review these instructions very carefully with our clients both initially and during subsequent weeks when training on using the *Weekly Record* is ongoing.

Because the self-monitoring of panic is so critical to clinical strategies, several issues reflecting recent developments in research clinics around the world are worth noting. First, as mentioned, it is clear that it is unsatisfactory to ask for reports of panic retrospectively—that is, "How many panic attacks have you had for the last 3 days or the last week, or the last month?" A clinician must use prospective self-monitoring of some type. Second, it has become apparent that simple recording of frequency of panic results in an extremely variable record that is often inadequate for data analysis and probably misleading clinically. What happens, for example, is that clients often, after becoming sensitive to what is a panic and what is not, correctly record less intensive "bursts" of anxiety as panic attacks. This results in little or no change in frequency over time. Panic attacks might also decrease considerably in duration. These less intense, shorter "panics" comprise the "rumblings" that usually remain to some extent in clients even after successful drug or behavioral treatment. At this point, clients have difficulty deciding whether this is a true "panic," resulting in wide variability from day to day in the same client or among clients in frequency of panic.

Alternatively, a client might decide that only the most severe burst (8 on a scale of 0 to 8) qualifies for panic and not record somewhat less intense instances of panic, thereby providing a misleading picture. Occasionally, these definitions may change from week to week in the mind of the same client. Therefore, several centers, including ours, have chosen to record self-monitored panic in a frequency $\times$ intensity $\times$ duration multiple. This results in what seems to be a more valid and satisfactory measure that eliminates the extreme variability and reflects clinical reality.

A Note on Physiological Assessment

The assessment of physiological responding is of theoretical as well as practical interest and until recently has been considered an essential component by many in the assessment of clinical anxiety. Recent data collected in our clinic, however, have changed our thinking somewhat on the usefulness of physiological assessment as a measure of clinical change (Barlow, 1988; Holden & Barlow, 1986). Although physiological assessment may have other equally important uses that are not necessarily connected with clinical change, we do not at this time recommend routine assessment of physiological responding for clinical purposes.

4

Introduction to the Treatment of Panic Disorder: Session 1

Overview

In this chapter we introduce the basic format and schedule for our panic treatment program. In each of the next three chapters we present one of the major components of the treatment program in a detailed protocol format. While we conceptualize our panic treatment as having three individual components, we also consider it a total treatment package that is presented to the clients in an integrated and coordinated fashion. The three major components of the treatment package include two anxiety management techniques—relaxation training and cognitive-behavior therapy—and the core treatment component—exposure therapy.

Because we are just now in the process of dismantling this treatment package in order to evaluate the relative contribution of each of the treatment components, we are not yet in a position to describe accurately either the relative contributions of the three components or the particular mechanisms that the components exert in the treatment of panic disorder. On the other hand, we do have substantial data (see Chapter 2) that support the use and utility of the treatment package as a whole. Although in actual practice the three treatment components are presented in an integrated fashion, for the purposes of this manual we have decided to present each of the components in a separate chapter. In so doing, the distinction among the three components is made clearer, and it allows the reader to select which of the components he/she may wish to use in his/her own treatment protocol. We feel this flexibility will allow clinicians to select the management skills that are most appropriate for any individual client. On the other hand, it does mean that the reader may have to combine protocol or session elements from two or more chapters in order to present the integrated package as we normally do in our own clinic.

The format for each of the 15 sessions in the treatment package is presented in three major sections. The first section of each treatment session lists the specific goals established for that session. The second section lists the procedures that are to be presented during the treatment session. The third section of the format is what we call the review and planning part of the session. For each of these format sections, detailed instructions and rationales are provided for the therapist. In addition, we occasionally include what we call "therapist reminders," which are practical notes to the therapist that cover a range of topics related to the procedures for a particular session. The final chapter of the book includes a case example in which the techniques and procedures outlined for the 15 sessions are provided.

Throughout the treatment protocol, we provide suggested scripts in order to present examples of how the content of the treatment protocol might be presented to clients. We strongly suggest that the reader see these merely as *examples* of how the content might be provided rather than as scripts that are to be presented to the client verbatim. That is, we recommend that the therapist attempt to present to clients the content of the protocol within the therapist's own clinical style and in a fashion that is most suitable for the client. Thus, we consider this to be a treatment protocol that is to be used by experienced clinicians who have some background in dealing with anxiety disorder cases. Some components of this treatment package require a great deal of experience with some of the procedures used in the protocol; for example, the cognitive protocol requires experience and training in the use of cognitive therapy techniques.

The practicalities of conducting the panic treatment surely are familiar to all clinicians. However, in order to make this as complete a treatment protocol as possible, we also mention a few general procedures. In our clinic we use a SOAP format (Subject data, Objective data, Assessment of data, Planning) (Ryback, Longabaugh, & Fowler, 1981) for writing all progress notes and client contacts. While other methods for writing progress notes are available and perhaps just as useful, we find the SOAP procedure, because of its structure and standardization, a convenient and efficient way to ensure consistency among therapists at the clinic.

As with any treatment program, it is extremely important to emphasize to the client the importance of accurate and consistent data collection during the whole treatment program. In this particular treatment package the accurate and consistent collection of data is especially important because the data that the client provides are incorporated into and provide a basis for developing some of the treatment strategies used in the protocol.

Every clinician is well aware of the kinds of scheduling difficulties that develop in the course of providing any kind of treatment. In order to help alleviate or to avoid unexpected difficulties in scheduling appointments, starting from the very first session we make clear to the client what the treatment schedule is. That is, we tell the clients that there will be 15 weekly sessions that will last approximately 60 minutes per session. We encourage clients to look ahead on their calendars and to schedule their appointments as well as possible. While we recognize that events may occur requiring changes of appointments, we make it clear that should an appointment need to be cancelled, it should be cancelled at least 24 hours in advance except under emergency conditions. The schedule of treatment sessions and the procedures that are presented in each session in the integrated protocol are presented in Table 4-1.

The remainder of this chapter presents the treatment protocol for the first treatment session. Basically, in the first session we introduce the treatment to the client and provide a rationale for and a detailed schedule of the treatment program. We also deal with any idiosyncratic practicalities (e.g., scheduling problems) that may have to be facilitated. Because this is a general introductory session, some of the content provided in this chapter overlaps slightly with some of the content that is presented again in later chapters in the treatment protocol. We have found, however, that a bit of redundancy in the treatment protocol may, in fact, be somewhat facilitative because the client's anticipation and generally elevated anxiety levels during the first couple of therapy sessions sometimes make it difficult for him/her to fully comprehend or understand the rationales in the procedures that are going to be used throughout the rest of the treatment program. We should also like to remind the reader that by the time the client arrives for the first therapy session at our clinic, he/she has already completed at least one thorough diagnostic interview and a complete assessment package that includes questionnaires and in some instances a psychophysiological examination. Thus, the therapist enters the therapy situation with a good deal of information about the client, and, of course, the client is at least generally familiar with the overall operation and procedures of our clinic.

TABLE 4-1. Schedule of Treatment Sessions for the Integrated Panic Treatment Protocol

Session	Exposure procedure	Relaxation procedure	Cognitive procedure
1	Introduction and treatment rationale	Present rationale and data-collection techniques	Present rationale
2		16-muscle-group relaxation	Introduce techniques for monitoring cognitions
3		16-muscle-group relaxation with discrimination training	Present didactic material on exploring alternatives
4		8-muscle-group relaxation with discrimination training	Introduce analysis of faulty logic
5		8-muscle-group relaxation training	Present didactic material on: a. decatastrophizing b. rescue factors c. reattribution d. hypothesis testing
6	Develop exposure hierarchy	4-muscle-group relaxation training	Begin imaginary practice for covert rehearsal
7	Imaginal exposure and panic symptom induction; breathing training	4-muscle-group relaxation training	Hypothesis testing and cognitive coping strategy practice
8	Imaginal exposure and self-exposure homework	4-muscle-group relaxation training by recall	Hypothesis testing, thought stopping, and diversionary techniques for anxiety management
9	Imaginal exposure and self-exposure homework	Relaxation by recall	Hypothesis testing and cognitive management practice
10	Imaginal exposure and self-exposure homework	Cue-controlled relaxation	Hypothesis testing and cognitive management practice
11	Imaginal exposure and self-exposure homework	Cue-controlled relaxation	Hypothesis testing and cognitive management practice

TABLE 4-1. (continued)

Session	Exposure procedure	Relaxation procedure	Cognitive procedure
12	Imaginal exposure and self-exposure homework	Generalization practice	Hypothesis testing and cognitive management practice
13	Generalization practice	Generalization practice	Generalization practice
14	Generalization practice	Generalization practice	Generalization practice
15	Generalization practice and termination issues	Generalization practice and termination issues	Generalization practice and termination issues

Treatment Session 1: Introduction to the Treatment of Panic Disorder

A. Session Goals

1. Introduce the client to the therapist.
2. Give description of the treatment program.
3. Give rationale for the treatment program.
4. Schedule treatment (once a week for the next 15 weeks).
5. Emphasize the importance of keeping accurate records and of practicing regularly.
6. Assess treatment credibility with questionnaire.

Therapist Reminder. As you begin the panic treatment protocol with your clients, there are several points to keep in mind. Remind your client of the schedule of appointments. This schedule requires that the client be seen once a week for 15 weeks. Also, tell the client that treatment sessions will take about 60 minutes.

At each session it will be important to collect *Weekly Records* and practice records to check to see that these sheets are being filled in correctly, to check to see how the person is getting along generally, to see if keeping the *Weekly Record* has led the client to discover anything about his/her anxiety, and to be supportive and empathetic, all in the service of maintaining a good therapeutic relationship.

B. Session Procedures

1. RATIONALE

Spend the initial 5 minutes with general introductions and then begin with a general inquiry into the client's primary anxiety problems. Indicate that while the client has already provided a great deal of information during the initial assessments, you would like to begin by having the client tell you personally some of his/her main difficulties.

Then focus on identifying the pattern of anxiety and particularly try to get the client to identify situations in which anxiety and panic attacks are more likely to occur. This may require some careful questioning and some degree of persistence. Many clients will be able readily to identify specific antecedents of anxiety but some clients are likely to have some difficulty, feeling that anxiety can occur at almost any time and that there does not seem to be any relationship between environmental situations or stressors and the occurrence of anxiety. For these clients in particular (but for all clients as well), you should attempt to identify any internal cues that may trigger anxiety. These internal cues might involve physical sensations or symptoms, negative verbal cognitions, and/or catastrophic imagery. Equal importance should be given to somatic, environmental, and cognitive cues.

Explain that you will be presenting information to the client about anxiety—what it is and how it functions—and about panic disorder in particular. The following text provides an example of the information that may be presented to clients during the first session.

Panic disorder is one of six types of anxiety problems that generally are recognized as distinct disorders by psychologists and psychiatrists. Overall, the anxiety disorders are quite common, appearing in over 10% of the general adult population. Anxiety problems also account for a large number of visits to general medical practitioners. While anxiety is a central feature of all these disorders, each of the disorders has other features that distinguish it from the rest. In simple phobias, the person is inordinately anxious, but only when confronted with a particular situation. For example, acrophobia is a fear of heights; the acrophobic becomes very anxious when in a precariously high perch, but otherwise is not usually bothered by the anxiety.

In the case of panic disorder, you are troubled by panic attacks and the haunting fear that another attack may occur at any time. During a panic attack, there is a sudden rush of anxiety that reaches its peak in anywhere from a few seconds to several minutes. We believe that because of the fear associated with panic attacks, some people begin to avoid situations or activities in which they have had panic attacks, and panickers develop what we call anticipatory anx-iety—that is, anxiety or fear that another panic attack will occur.

The symptoms that occur during a panic attack are the same body responses that occur naturally when a person is faced with an emergency or life-threatening situation. These body responses prepare one to react and deal with the emergency by either fleeing or taking some other action. In this sense, then, panic attacks may be thought of as a hard-wired automatic fear response in its most pure form. In the presence of a threatening cue or situation, this panic-fear response is helpful and serves as a naturally occurring "body alarm" that signals danger. On the other hand, if the alarm goes off at times other than a real threat situation, it is a false alarm. Unfortunately, our body still responds as if it were a "real alarm."

While we are not yet sure why or how these false alarms occur, false alarms are generally accompanied by the same body responses associated with a "real alarm" (such as heart rate increase). Further, stressful events may lead to an increase in one or more of those body responses associated with alarm. We believe that through a learning process called interoceptive conditioning these physical cues become associated with full-blown alarms and come to serve as signals to initiate a false alarm. Thus, whenever heart rate or breathing rate (or probably a whole host of body responses) reaches a critical level, it comes to initiate the panic attack. Because stressful events are likely to lead to these body responses, panic attacks are more likely in stressful situations.

In addition, because the experience of these false alarms is unpleasant, we come to dread the possibility of another one occurring. We have labeled the worry and concern about having a false alarm "anticipatory anxiety." Because anticipatory anxiety itself is stressful, it, too, helps produce the same body responses that may lead to panic attacks. In some cases people begin to avoid situations in which panic attacks have occurred in order to help control their anxiety or to help reduce the number or type of stressful situations in which they expose themselves.

In any case, anxiety is an emotion that is experienced by every single individ-ual. Anxiety is part of the experience of being human. Anxiety is not necessarily always bad, but in some individuals it can occur either excessively frequently and/ or at extreme levels of intensity so that it is distressing and it can interfere with the individual's level of functioning. In cases such as these, professional help is frequently necessary in order to help the client understand anxiety, reduce the frequency and/or level of anxiety, and learn how to deal better with stress as well as anxiety itself so that there is less likelihood of problems in the future.

Tell me again, how do you know when you're anxious? What are some of the things you feel, think, and do? (*The therapist should allow time for a response.*) When individuals with anxiety problems talk about anxiety, they usually mention a wide variety of physical feelings or symptoms as well as negative feelings and thoughts, and sometimes changes in behavior. The individual may report feeling tense, nervous, noticing rapid pulse, having difficulty breathing, frequent or excessive sweating, butterflies in the stomach, etcetera. Clients also report feelings of impending doom, thoughts that something terrible is about to happen, and a great deal of worrying and brooding about the present and particularly their future. Sometimes, clients also report changes in behavior associated with anxiety. These behavioral changes may include disruption of performance, such as when anxiety interferes with one's ability to do a good job in work or to complete a necessary task, and sometimes may include avoiding certain places or situations. In fact, researchers have agreed that with most clients, anxiety seems to be an emotion that consists of a combination of three variables: physiological, cognitive, and behavioral. Some individuals may be more aware of the physical side of anxiety whereas other clients may be more aware of the cognitive or behavioral side of anxiety. For most individuals who are participating in this treatment program, the physiological and cognitive components of anxiety appear to be most disturbing. However, all three aspects probably play some role in the experience of anxiety for almost all individuals with anxiety problems. Therefore, our treatment program will include procedures designed to work on all of these aspects of anxiety.

You then should elaborate further on our model of anxiety. First, you can discuss the physiological apsects of anxiety:

Anxiety involves increased physiological arousal of the autonomic nervous system. The autonomic nervous system is that part of the nervous system that controls many of our bodily processes or bodily activities, particularly the functioning of the internal organs, such as the cardiovascular and gastrointestinal systems. When an individual experiences high levels of anxiety, some of the bodily processes are automatically increased. For example, blood flow to the extremities such as the hands, arms, and legs, may be increased while blood flow to the head and to the internal organs will be decreased. The individual's heart and breathing rate may become more rapid while digestion may be slowed down. Thus, anxiety is not just something that is "all in the individual's head," but rather does involve some real physical changes. There is increased physiological arousal in at least some of the body's organs. Many of these physical changes also occur during exercise, excitement, sexual arousal, etcetera.

This arousal is associated with a variety of sensations, feelings, or "symptoms" that are sometimes experienced by the individual as frightening or distressing. These sensations include familiar sensations of increased heart rate, dizziness, tingling of the fingers or the hand, difficulty breathing, feeling faint, and a wide variety of other symptoms. These sensations are all a result of the increased physiological arousal of the emotion of anxiety. They indeed can be quite unpleasant and distressing.

However, they are just sensations and they are not necessarily dangerous. Anxiety involves an exaggeration of normal bodily processes. Everybody probably experiences at least some of the physical sensations or symptoms of anxiety at least occasionally. Some people actually go out of their way to experience these sensations—for example, by riding roller coasters, watching suspense or horror movies. As stated before, however, some individuals experience these sensations more frequently or at higher levels. However, again it is important to recognize that anxiety involves normal bodily reactions. The higher frequency or intensity of anxiety can be reduced by certain treatment procedures that will be part of the treatment program. We discuss these treatments more later.

The second major aspect of anxiety is what we have already described as the cognitive component, or the component involving our thoughts, beliefs, expectations, and so on. All persons are influenced greatly by the type of things that we think about and the evaluations, interpretations, or appraisals of experiences. In short, our thoughts influence our moods, feelings, and behaviors. We frequently feel that our moods are determined by things that happen to us, our past experiences, situations we currently experience, etcetera.

For example, if a person says something to you that is insulting, that you feel is insulting, you might react by saying, "He/she made me feel angry." In actuality, however, people do not respond directly to situations that they experience; we really respond to the interpretations or evaluations associated with our experiences. For example, if someone says something is insulting to you, you could interpret that behavior as reflecting his/her immaturity or his/her own personal problems and decide that it is not necessary to become upset about it, that there is no need to feel insulted or hurt or to feel that you must "get back at" him/her in some way.

As another example (*The therapist can illustrate this to the client.*), if I were to point the pencil at you, you would be relatively unlikely to become upset or anxious. However, if I were to tell you that the pencil was really a pistol, it is quite likely that you would respond by becoming anxious, frightened, or perhaps angry. This is because you have interpreted the situation involving the gun as a dangerous situation, whereas the situation involving the pointing of the pencil is not interpreted as dangerous. If you didn't know that the pencil was a gun, you would not become anxious.

In a similar fashion, people label their experiences almost constantly. Unfortunately, at times, individuals' interpretations of situations and experiences do not seem to be that accurate or at least not that useful. Our interpretations can get in the way and can cause a considerable amount of problems.

For example, if a person interprets a brief conversation with a member of the opposite sex as one in which he/she made a bad impression by saying or doing something "wrong," he/she is likely to feel anxious, perhaps foolish, etcetera. It really isn't the social situation that resulted in the individual feeling anxious or embarrassed but that person's interpretation of the situation.

Our interpretations of situations can sometimes be identified or recognized by the type of things we say in various situations. We are now talking about the thoughts that the individual has. We use the term "self-statements" to refer to thoughts or types of things people talk about. Just as cognitions or interpretations or self-statements can bring on negative mood and negative feelings, they can be turned around or modified to improve our ability to cope with stress and to deal more productively with various experiences and situations. Part of the procedures we focus on during the treatment program consist of procedures for learning different ways of dealing cognitively with stress and anxiety.

The third major component of anxiety is the behavioral component. Anxiety may disrupt a person's performance, particularly for behaviors that require concentration or skill, such as reading, doing a job that is difficult, or presenting a speech. Anxiety can influence behavior in another way. Some persons learn to avoid situations or places in which they have experienced anxiety or where they think they might experience anxiety. We call this *avoidance behavior*. Or some persons may leave or run away from where they are when they start to experience anxiety. We call this *escape behavior*.

In general, persons in this treatment program don't have much problem with avoidance or escape. They tend to try to continue to go wherever they have to go to try to "stick it out" when anxiety occurs, rather than avoiding or escaping. This is a good approach, and we encourage you to continue going places as much as you can. If you do have any problems avoiding or escaping from places, please let me know and we may decide to work on these problems too.

A more common problem among persons in this program is that they may often adopt a "spectator role" in situations where they experience anxiety. That is, they become so occupied with their level of anxiety or their negative thoughts that they divert their attention away from the task at hand, and this in turn results in inefficiency. For example, an individual may become so preoccupied with the impression he/she is making in a social situation that he/she actually misses parts of the conversation.

Persons with generalized anxiety and panic disorders often do report that their anxiety does interfere with their performance. The treatment strategies you'll be learning are designed to reduce anxiety and to help you cope better with anxiety that does occur. These strategies, therefore, are likely to decrease the extent to which anxiety interferes with or disrupts your behavior and performance.

To briefly review, there are three major components of anxiety.

• First, the physiological arousal that is associated with different physical sensations or feelings.

• Second, the cognitive component, which involves our thoughts or self-statements and our beliefs, interpretations, and expectations, as well as our visual imagery.

• Third, overt behavior, including avoidance and escape responses and quality of performance of skills and tasks.

It seems quite clear that these three components of anxiety are frequently related to one another. Increase in anxiety may predispose a person to panic attacks—that is, false alarms—just as stress generally seems to be related to panic attacks. At times, conditions may bring about increased physical arousal, which is then interpreted as anxiety, which may then interfere with overt behavior. Alternatively, sometimes people respond to physical sensations by interpreting them as signs of anxiety, which increases the likelihood of feeling even more anxious.

Remember, as I stated just a few minutes ago, the various physical sensations of anxiety are due to various changes in physiological arousal and are natural bodily changes that may be unpleasant but that are not dangerous. However, these can be seen as stimuli or events that can be interpreted by the individual. In many cases, the individual interprets or labels these physical sensations as being in some way extremely dangerous or terrifying or the worst thing that could happen.

For example, an individual who is sensitized to the experience of anxiety may be aware of any changes in their bodily feelings. Any time that they identify some increased level of physical arousal, such as a more rapid heart rate, they interpret these changes as meaning that maybe they are going to die, faint, or somehow lose control. This is an interpretation of physical changes. The interpretation is not necessarily correct and is quite likely to be very frightening. The fear may then become associated with the physical or environmental cue. Thus the erroneous interpretation increases the individual's likelihood of experiencing anxiety. This increased anxiety may then result in even higher levels of physical arousal or physical sensations, which then in turn may result in greater worries about personal health, sanity, or ability to remain in control of him/herself. Thus, a vicious cycle has been established, in which physical sensations increase the likelihood of further physical arousal, more negative thinking, and greater experience of the emotion of anxiety.

2. EXPLANATION OF TREATMENT

Now I'd like to talk a little bit more about the specifics of the treatment program. Our treatment program consists of relaxation training, cognitive techniques, and exposure therapy, each of which is designed to teach you how to change your reactions to stress and false alarms. The relaxation skills will help you change your physical (somatic) reactions to stress, and the cognitive techniques are aimed at changing the worrisome thoughts that often accompany stress reactions. We think of these procedures as ways to manage anxiety and to increase the likelihood of your completing the exposure therapy.

In vivo exposure is our term for confronting directly in real-life situations the cues that might set off false alarms and teaching yourself how to respond differently to those cues. We also use imaginal exposure in which you visualize the panic provoking cues that increase your anxiety. These treatments have been shown to be effective for anxiety and panic problems. After you learn to master these treatment procedures, you will be much better able to understand anxiety, to deal with stress and to reduce anxiety in a wide range of situations. We will begin learning the actual coping strategies next week. As I have already explained, anxiety in certain situations may be caused either by your physical reactions, your interpretations of the reactions, or by what you say to yourself in stressful situations.

The first few sessions of this treatment will be devoted largely to training beginning relaxation skills, but you will also begin to monitor your thinking in stressful situations. We'll also begin to discuss several types of thinking that typically lead to anxiety. As you become more proficient in relaxation skills and begin to practice relaxation strategies more easily, less treatment time will be devoted to relaxation training and more time will be spent on learning cognitive coping techniques.

As you become more proficient with these management skills, you will begin to use them in real-life situations. We feel strongly that the most therapeutic experiences for you will be the *in vivo* exposures. Because we are going to be asking you to confront and cope with anxiety provoking situations, both in your imagination as well as in reality, we expect that you might find yourself becoming more anxious before you start feeling better. In fact, we look for these increases in anxiety as a temporary marker suggesting that our clients are doing what is necessary for them to improve.

Our experience with this treatment package has shown that when patients complete the program and practice regularly, they improve substantially by the end of treatment and they continue to improve even after treatment ends.

Do you have any questions? Then we'll begin the relaxation training at your next session.

C. Review and Planning

As I stated earlier, practice is essential for you to receive major benefit from the treatment. It is also important to remember that it will take some time before you feel more relaxed in general. You have probably been very tense and nervous for quite a while, and it will take a while to learn to cope with your anxiety. You will gradually become more aware of your level of tension during the day. You can use the ability to relax and to change your thoughts as active coping tactics when you begin to experience anxiety.

Give the client new *Weekly Records* and review the one he/she has filled out for the preceding week or two. Given any suggestions for correct completion of the records. Again, emphasize the need to keep accurate records. You may want to role-play a panic episode to give the client some supervised practice in filling out the *Weekly Record*. Again, remind the client of the treatment schedule and the importance of keeping accurate data because those data will provide important information to tailor treatment to the client's specific needs.

5

Relaxation Treatment Component

Learning how to relax has long been considered a "common sense" method for coping with stress, anxiety, and anger. Folklore advises that when faced with a stressful or anger arousing situation simply "take a deep breath and slowly count to ten" before acting. The logic of this advice, at least implicitly, recognizes that these emotional situations lead to excessive levels of physiological arousal that may interfere with adequate coping responses. The negative affective state associated with the arousal and associated action tendencies, in its most general sense, has been labeled *anxiety*.

The role of residual tension (i.e., the neuromuscular tension remaining when an individual simply lies still and attempts to relax) and its relationship to both behavior and emotional states was first described and studied by Jacobson (1938). In these early and important studies Jacobson showed that induction of a deep state of relaxation does in fact attenuate various reflexive responses as well as improving mental activities and reducing emotional reactions, including reactions to sudden pain. Later studies have substantiated Jacobson's early work and have shown that patients who display chronic anxiety and/or other forms of anxiety disorders have higher levels of resting baseline muscle tension and autonomic activity than do nonpatient controls (Barlow, 1988). Subsequent to Jacobson's work, Wolpe (1958) incorporated relaxation techniques into his method of systematic desensitization. Thus, the common sense of folklore turns out not only to be an effective treatment method for anxiety problems but in fact has been scientifically substantiated.

In a review of the relaxation training research, Hillenberg and Collins (1982) found that practice in relaxation skills has been successfully applied to a wide variety of problems, including sleep disturbances, headache, hypertension, general anxiety, test anxiety, speech anxiety, hyperactivity, asthma, drinking behavior, and anger control. In addition, a large number of clinical analogue studies (e.g., Borkovec, Grayson, & Cooper, 1978) have found that training in relaxation skills does reduce tension in a variety of nonclinical populations. In many of these studies, reductions in tension and/or anxiety were measured by decreases in various physiological responses, including skeletal muscle tension, blood pressure, heart rate, pulse pressure, or various combinations of these measures.

Few studies have directly assessed different treatment programs for panic disorder. But several research programs (Waddell, Barlow, & O'Brien, 1984; Cerny *et al.*, 1984; Gitlan *et al.*, 1985) have incorporated relaxation training into multicomponent treatment programs, presumably to help cope with the somatic complaints associated with panic disorder. But the process of training panic patients to relax has its own potential advantages as well as pitfalls.

The pitfalls include the well-established phenomenon of relaxation-induced anxiety (RIA) (Heide & Borkovec, 1984) and relaxation-induced panic (RIP) (Adler, Craske, & Barlow, 1987). It is not unusual for panic patients to become anxious or even panic when first attempting relaxation, particularly at home away from the therapist. Procedures described in this chapter are designed to minimize that possibility, but if it does occur, it can be turned to a therapeutic advantage. Specifically, disturbances in physiological homeostasis occasioned by relaxation may provide a set of interoceptive cues associated with panic (panic cues). Thus, relaxation itself becomes yet another occasion for exposure to panic cues (see Chapter 7) and an opportunity to practice coping responses conveyed during the course of treatment. Most often, RIA or RIP passes quickly if it occurs under therapeutic guidance.

The relaxation training component for our panic treatment program is based largely on Bernstein and Borkovec's (1973) procedure for progressive relaxation training. The Bernstein and Borkovec program represents both a refinement and a modification of Jacobson's (1938) method of progressive relaxation. For the most part, we have followed the procedures described by Bernstein and Borkovec; however, the procedure that we use in our panic treatment program has been modified in the following ways:

1. We use 12 to 14 relaxation training sessions, as opposed to the 10 sessions recommended in Bernstein and Borkovec.

2. The sequence of muscle groups described by Bernstein and Borkovec are altered to go from hands and arms to feet and legs and thence up the body to the face and forehead.

3. Tensing of the chest is done by having the client take a deep breath and hold it.

4. The shoulders and the lower back are tensed separately rather than together.

5. We use counting to deepen relaxation from the beginning of the training program rather than as an ancillary method introduced only in later sessions.

6. We include discrimination training as originally recommended by Jacobson (1938) at several points throughout the training program.

7. Clients are encouraged to practice using the relaxation skills to cope with anxiety that is generated by visualizing anxiety reactions or by other anxiety-induction techniques (see Chapters 6 and 7).

All of the preceding procedural modifications were based on research or the clinical experience of the authors and other personnel at the Center for Stress and Anxiety Disorders. Most of these additions have been shown to be effective modifications of the basic progressive relaxation training procedure (Canter, Kondo, & Knott, 1975; Hutchings, Denney, Basgall, & Houston, 1980; Raskin, Bali, & Peeke, 1980). Because this program is a treatment package that integrates three treatment components, we have incorporated structured rehearsal of relaxation skills (see Item 7 above) during therapy sessions. The procedures for structured rehearsal were modeled after Suinn's (1977) anxiety management techniques (see Denney, 1980; Hutchings *et al.*, 1980).

The remainder of this chapter is a detailed description of the progressive relaxation training program used in our panic treatment package. The training procedure is described on a session-by-session basis over the course of the 15-session treatment program. Though we present the relaxation training procedure separately from other components of the treatment program, we remind the reader that the relaxation training component is only one of the three major components involved in the panic treatment program and as such is integrated with the other components throughout the treatment protocol. Generally speaking, we attempt to place heavier emphasis on relaxation training early in the treatment protocol and devote less time to relaxation training later in the treatment protocol as the client becomes more skilled in relaxation training. In later sessions, we also introduce the structured rehearsal of relaxation skills. These structured practices are presented along with cognitive strategies as a means of dealing with anxiety and panicky feelings induced by imagination or other means (e.g., physical exertion) during treatment sessions. The specifics of the anxiety-induction procedures are presented in Chapter 7. The treatment rationale and basic therapy instructions, which comprise the first treatment session, were presented in Chapter 4, along with the exact schedule for relaxation training. Thus, we begin with Session 2 in this chapter.

Session 2

A. Session Goals

1. Discuss episodes of heightened anxiety that have occurred since the last session.
2. Begin to identify antecedents to the anxiety.
3. Show the client how to tense the muscles for relaxation training.
4. Go through 16-muscle-group training and give the client a practice tape.
5. Show the client how to record practices on the *Relaxation Practice Record* (see Appendix C; "practice record"). This is described more fully in Chapter 8.

B. Session Procedures

1. Review the *Weekly Record* with the client. Discuss any episodes of heightened anxiety, and begin to have the client try to identify specific antecedents to his/her anxiety. Inquire as to how the client handles these situations. Tell the client that he/she will be learning both to become more aware of tension/anxiety at earlier stages and to respond differently to these situations by relaxing.
2. Introduce relaxation training.

As we discussed previously, this treatment program is focused on the behavioral, cognitive, and physiological components of panic disorder. The behavioral component refers to avoidance and escape responses as well as the performance of any skill or task. The cognitive component involves our thoughts or self-statements, our beliefs, interpretations, expectations, and imagery. The physiological component is associated with different physical sensations or feelings.

It seems quite clear that these three components of anxiety are frequently related to one another. At times, cognitions may bring about increased physical arousal, which is then interpreted as anxiety, which may then interfere with overt behavior. Alternatively, sometimes persons respond to physical sensations by interpreting them as signs of anxiety, which increases the likelihood of feeling even more anxious.

The various physical sensations of anxiety are due to various changes in physiological arousal and are natural bodily changes that may be unpleasant but that are not dangerous. These bodily changes can be seen as stimuli or events that can be interpreted by the individual. In many cases, the individual interprets or labels these physical sensations as being in some way extremely dangerous or terrifying or the worst thing that could happen.

For example, an individual who is sensitized to the experience of anxiety may be aware of any changes in their bodily feelings. Any time that the person identifies some increased level of physical arousal, such as a more rapid heart rate, the person interprets these changes as meaning that maybe he/she is going to die, faint, or somehow lose control. This is an interpretation of physical changes. The interpretation is not necessarily correct, and it is quite likely to be very frightening. Thus, this erroneous interpretation of bodily changes increases the individual's experiences of anxiety. This increased anxiety may then result in even higher levels of physical arousal or physical sensations, which in turn may result in greater worries about the person's health, sanity, or ability to remain in control of him/herself. Thus, a vicious cycle has been established, in which physical sensations increase the likelihood of further physical arousal, more negative thinking, and greater experience of the emotion of anxiety.

The treatment component you are beginning now is designed to help you learn to decrease the unpleasant physical symptoms, muscle tension, and anxiety that you experience.

This component of the treatment program consists of relaxation training. Relaxation training has been shown to be an effective technique for managing anxiety. Let me explain the treatment in more detail to you now.

Relaxation training consists of the systematic tensing and relaxation of the major muscle groups of the whole body. After going through this series of tension–relaxation exercises or cycles, most people feel relaxed. With practice, and I want to emphasize the word *practice*, one can learn to become deeply relaxed fairly rapidly. Obviously, it is impossible to be tense and relaxed at the same time. You can learn how to relax and use this skill when you notice that you are becoming tense and anxious.

Achieving a state of deep relaxation is a learned skill, somewhat like learning to ride a bicycle. To be really effective, one must practice regularly. Also, as you practice, you should begin to be more aware of the tension in your body, to be able to recognize it earlier, and to localize it so that it becomes something with which you can more readily cope.

For this training to be of the most benefit to you, you should go through the exercises for about 20 minutes, twice per day. If you cannot find time for two practices per day, one is acceptable but not as good as twice per day. If you cannot, or will not, practice regularly, then you probably will not receive the major benefits of the training program.

3. Initial 16-muscle-group training.

a. First, you should point to the muscle groups on your own body as you list the 16 muscle groups. The muscle groups are as follows:

Muscle group number	Body parts
1, 2	Hand and lower arm, right, left, then both together
3, 4	Upper arm, right, left, then both together
5, 6	Lower leg and foot, right, left, then both together
7	Thighs
8	Abdomen
9	Chest and breathing
10, 11	Shoulders and lower neck
12	Back of neck
13	Lips
14	Eyes
15	Lower forehead
16	Upper forehead

b. Next, show the client how to tense each muscle group. While we have found the following procedures to be quite successful, others may be used.

• *Lower arm*—Make fist, palm down, and pull wrist up toward upper arm.

• *Upper arm*—Tense biceps. With arms by side, pull upper arm toward side without touching. (Try not to tense lower arm while doing this, let lower arm hang loosely.)

• *Lower leg and foot*—Extend leg so it's straight. Point toe upward toward knees.

• *Thighs*—Pull knees together until upper legs feel tense.

• *Abdomen*—Pull in stomach toward back.

• *Chest and breathing*—Take a deep breath and hold it about 10 seconds then release.

• *Shoulders and lower neck*—Shrug shoulders, then bring shoulders up until they touch ears.

• *Back of neck*—Put head back and press against back of chair.

• *Lips*—Press lips together: don't clench teeth or jaw.

• *Eyes*—Close eyes tightly but don't close too hard (be careful if you have contact lenses).

• *Lower forehead*—Pull eyebrows down (try to get them to meet).

• *Upper forehead*—Raise eyebrows and wrinkle your forehead.

Tell the client to keep his/her eyes closed during the entire training session. Help the client repeat the sequence of muscle groups in order to assure that the client understands what the muscle group sequence will be.

Next, you should demonstrate the relaxation procedure, using your right lower arm. Then you will ask the client to tense his/her right hand and lower arm, to attend to the sensations of tension in that arm, and then to relax it. When most clients relax the hand and arm, they will not relax the whole arm from the shoulders down. Therefore, ask the client to try again and when he/she relaxes, really let the muscles go completely limp so that the whole arm from the shoulder all the way down can become relaxed. You can support the patient's arm and show them what you mean. Repeat this until he/she completely relaxes on instruction.

Next, tell the client that you will be instructing him/her to tense the various muscle groups you have mentioned, that you will be calling attention to the sensations she/he is probably experiencing and giving various other suggestions. Once more, assist the client in repeating the muscle-group sequence. The client should remove eyeglasses (if worn) and loosen very restrictive clothing such as jackets, shoes, and so on. You may wish to dim the room lights at this point. The goal is to help the client become as comfortable as possible before beginning the relaxation training.

Next, go through the aforementioned muscle groups. Have the client (1) tense the muscle groups for 5 to 10 seconds, (2) attend to the sensations of tension in that particular muscle group and area of the body, (3) relax the muscle, and (4) notice the difference between the tension and the relaxation. For the limbs, do right lower arm and hand, then left lower arm and hand, and then the two together; right upper arm, left upper arm and the two together; right lower leg and foot, left lower leg and foot, and the two together. For all the others, you will not have this bilateral aspect. Between each muscle group, allow about 20 seconds with either a comment — "Just continue to relax" — or one of the suggestions for patter listed here later. This particular material includes suggestions for relaxation that may help; use these after every other tension–relaxation cycle and continue to cycle through the particular suggestions. There is no special magic to the particular wording, but try to use something approximating this content and with which you also feel comfortable. Go through the tension–relaxation exercises for all the muscle groups; this should probably take 20 minutes or so.

When all the tension–relaxation cycles have been completed, go through the deepening exercises by counting from 1 to 5. Tell the person you are going to count from 1 to 5 and that as you count, he/she will become more relaxed. Again, intersperse suggestions of greater relaxation between the numbers and try to time the counts to an expiration.

Once you have done the deepening suggestions, ask the person to concentrate on his/her breathing, to breathe through his/her nose, and to concentrate on his/her breathing. Suggest that as he/she breathes in, he/she can feel the cool air and as he/she exhales, he/she can feel the warm air. Finally, tell the client he/she should think to himself/herself the word "relax" as he/she exhales. Allow about 1 or 2 minutes for this exercise, and repeat the instructions at least once.

After that, go through the reverse of the deepening counting from 5 back to 1. Tell the person that you are going to do that and suggest to him/her that, as you count, he/she is becoming more alert and that at "2" he/she will open his/her eyes and at "1" he/she will be back at a normal state of alertfulness.

Have the person remain seated after the alerting, but sitting up, so that he/she is now in an upright seated position. For people who wear glasses, return them. You want to inquire first if he/she became relaxed at all; second, if there were any particular signs of residual tension; third, if there were any other noticeable sensations or other things he/she wants to talk about.

After this, prepare and give the client an instruction sheet that lists the muscle groups and the aforementioned practice sequence. Also ask the client to record in his/her *Relaxation Practice Record* ("practice record") when he/she practiced, the length of time, and the approximate time of day. Have the client try to rate how relaxed he/she became for each practice using 1 as not being relaxed or tense and 10 as being very relaxed. Tell the client that most people are able to follow the relaxation procedure at home easily, but that some people find it helpful at first to use an audiotape recording to cue them. Therefore, we give the client an audiotape to take with him/her. However, initially we suggest that the client try the relaxation exercise without using the tape. If the client needs to use the tape as a learning aid, he/she should do so, but remind the client that our goal is to learn the procedure without the use of the tape recording. In our clinic, we simply tape record one of our staff administering 16-muscle-group relaxation. We have found these tapes to be both efficient and instructive. Professionally prepared relaxation tapes are available from several commercial sources. Because of our concern with RIA and because several of our clients have reported untoward effects when using commercially prepared tapes, we prefer to make our own tapes.

SAMPLE INSTRUCTIONS

Intimations for Deepening Relaxation after Tension Exercises
Now I want you to relax all the muscles of your body; just let them become more and more relaxed. I am going to help you to achieve a deeper state of relaxation by counting from one to five. As I count you will feel yourself becoming more and more deeply relaxed; . . . farther and farther down into a deep restful state of complete relaxation. One . . . you are going to become more deeply relaxed. Two . . . deeper and deeper into a very relaxed state . . . Three . . . four . . . more and more relaxed . . . five. Completely relaxed.

Attention to Breathing
Now I want you to remain in your very relaxed state. . . . I want you to begin to attend just to your breathing. Breathe through your nose. Notice the cool air as you breathe in (*pair with inhalation*) . . . and the warm moist air as you exhale (*pair with exhalation*). . . . Just continue to attend to your breathing. . . . Now each time you exhale, mentally repeat the word "relax." Inhale, exhale, relax (*pair with respiratory cycle*). . . . Inhale, exhale, relax. . . .

Some clients may have difficulty with the cadence of the whole procedure. An alternative procedure is to match the first syllable of the word relax (*re-*) with inspiration and the second syllable (*-lax*) with expiration. While the first procedure is preferable, either seem to work satisfactorily if used correctly. The breathing practice should continue for at least 2 minutes.

Procedures for Alerting
Now I am going to help you to return to your normal state of alertfulness. In a little while, I shall begin counting backwards froms five to one. You will gradually become more alert. When I reach "two," I want you to open your eyes. When I get to "one," you will be entirely roused to your normal state of alertfulness. Ready now? Five . . . four . . . three . . . two. . . . Now your eyes are opened and you begin to feel very alert. Returning completely to your normal state . . . one. (*Pause 10 seconds.*)

Instructions during Tension–Relaxation Exercises
Now I want you to tense the muscles of your [muscle area] by [tensing instructions]. Study the tensions located in [tension location]. (*Pause.*)
(*After subject has tensed the muscle group for ten seconds:*) Now relax the muscles of your [muscle area], and study the differences betweens the tension and the relaxation.

Suggested Patter between Exercise Procedures

1. Just let yourself become more and more relaxed. If you feel yourself becoming drowsy, that will be fine too. As you think of relaxation and of letting go of your muscles, they will become more loose . . . heavy . . . relaxed. Just let your muscles go as you become more and more relaxed.

2. (*Pause 20 seconds.*)

3. You are becoming more and more relaxed, sleepy and relaxed, but you will not go to sleep. As you become more relaxed, you will feel yourself settling deep into the chair. All your muscles are becoming more and more comfortable relaxed . . . loose . . . heavy . . . and relaxed.

4. (*Pause 20 seconds.*)

5. The relaxation is growing deeper and still deeper. You are relaxed . . . drowsy and relaxed. Your breathing is regular and relaxed. With each breath you take in, your relaxation increases. And each time you exhale, you spread the relaxation throughout your body.

6. (*Pause 20 seconds.*)

7. Note the pleasant feelings of warmth and heaviness that are coming into your body as your muscles relax completely. You will always be clearly aware of what you are doing and what I am saying as you become more deeply relaxed.

8. (*Pause 20 seconds.*)

9. Now the very deep state of relaxation is moving through all the areas of your body. You are becoming more and more comfortably relaxed . . . drowsy and relaxed. You can feel the comfortable sensations of relaxation as you go into a deeper . . . and deeper state of relaxation.

10. (*Pause 20 seconds.*)

On completing the relaxation practice, show the client how to fill out the practice record and instruct him/her to complete this record throughout treatment. Give the client a relaxation tape that is to be used if necessary. Instruct the client to use the tape *only if needed* to learn the muscle groups and to allow proper time for the relaxation. Explain to the client that the goal is to learn to relax without the use of the tape. But in the beginning, some people find using the tape helpful while learning how to relax. As soon as possible, the use of the tape should be discontinued. In any case, the tape should be returned to the therapist no later than Session 4.

C. Review and Planning

1. Review the importance of practicing relaxation twice daily and of recording practices on the practice record.

As I stated earlier, practice is essential to receive major benefit from the treatment. It is also important to remember that it will take some time before you feel more relaxed in general. You have probably been very tense and nervous for quite a while and it will take a while to learn to relax your muscles. You will gradually become more aware of your level of tension during the day. You can use the ability to relax quickly as an active coping tactic when you begin to experience anxiety.

2. Give the client new *Weekly Record* sheets, and review those he/she has filled out for the past few weeks. Give any suggestions for correct completion of the records. Again, emphasize the need to keep accurate records.

Session 3

A. Session Goals

1. Review the *Weekly Record* sheets and practice records, and discuss progress/problems.
2. Do 16-muscle-group training and add discrimination training.
3. Emphasize importance of noticing tension early on, so the client can begin to relax/cope with the anxiety/tension at an earlier stage.

B. Session Procedures

1. Review the client's *Weekly Record* and check whether the client has been practicing the relaxation exercises as prescribed. Fill in any gaps in data on the *Weekly Record* and/or practice record. Deal with any difficulties associated with completing assignments or data collection. You should repeatedly, but gently, remind and urge the client to practice regularly because only with repeated practice will lasting effects be obtained. You should also reinforce the notion that benefits cannot be expected overnight, that relaxation is not like a drug, which may bring changes in minutes or hours: Instead it is usually a matter of weeks. Make this point especially if a client seems discouraged!
2. Repeat the 16-muscle-group training and *add* discrimination training.
   a. Rationale for discrimination training

Today we are going to repeat the 16-muscle-group relaxation exercise, only this time we are going to do it a little differently. This change in the technique will help you become more aware of the different levels of tension you may experience and enable you to detect tension before it reaches high levels. We call this procedure *discrimination training* because it will help you *discriminate*—that is, recognize different levels of tension. It is easier to counteract tension when it is at a low level. Therefore, recognizing low levels of tension is another step toward dealing effectively with tension.

    b. Awareness training

• First ask the client to close his/her eyes and tense the lower right arm in the usual fashion and then relax it.

• Second, instruct the client to tense the arm only *half as much* as the time before, to concentrate on these half-tensed muscle sensations, and then to relax the arm completely.

• Then ask the client to tense the arm only *half as much* as the last time, or only *one-fourth* of the usual level of tension, to concentrate on these sensations, and then to relax the arm completely.

    c. Have the client open his/her eyes and inquire as to whether he/she understood the idea: that there are different levels of muscle tension and that these different levels feel differently.

• If the client seems to understand, proceed to Step 4.

• If the client does not seem to understand, repeat the rationale in Item a and the steps in Item b and then inquire again.

    d. Tell the client that you will ask him/her to engage in some discrimination training with neck and facial muscles during the relaxation training because it is in these muscle groups that tension is often first noticed.

    e. Add the following discrimination training steps for muscle groups 12 (back of neck) and 14 (eyes):

• Full tension and relaxation
• Half tension and relaxation
• One-quarter tension and relaxation

Remind clients during this part of training to pay special attention to the sensations of tension and how they differ from full to one-quarter tension.

    f. It will also be good if you can time the "tension release" or "relax" instruction to coincide with expiration. If it does not quite fit, do not be too concerned, however.

    3. If there is any residual tension in any muscle group, do additional relaxation for that muscle group.

C. Review and Planning

    1. Review the *Weekly Record* and practice records.

    2. Remind the client to do discrimination training while practicing relaxation at home.

3. Remind the client to use the relaxation tape only if necessary. Also check to make sure the client is not rushing through the relaxation practices and that the client's pacing during the practices allows for complete relaxation between tension–relaxation cycles.

Session 4

A. Session Goals

1. Review records and discuss progress/problems—especially assess the client's awareness of muscle tension during the week and use of discrimination training during home practice.
2. Go through the 8-muscle-group tension–relaxation procedure with discrimination training, and begin home practice with the 8-muscle-group procedure with discrimination practice.
3. Get relaxation tape back from the client (if not already received in Session 3).

B. Session Procedures

1. Eight-muscle-group training. The 8 muscle groups are as in Bernstein and Borkovec (1973). Include discrimination training with muscle groups 6 (neck) and 7 (eyes), as in the previous session.
- Both arms (Have the client hold both arms out, slightly flexed at the elbows and tense hands, lower, and upper arms.)
- Both lower legs
- Abdomen
- Chest by deep breath
- Shoulders
- Back of neck
- Eyes
- Forehead
2. Introduce the 8-muscle-group variation by telling the client that you will be reducing the number of muscle groups as a step toward shortening the procedure and making it a tactic that is "more portable" and readily usable. Go through the muscle groups to be used, and demonstrate the lower-arm flexion position.
3. Extend the interval between tension–relaxation cycles to at least 30 seconds.

4. At the end of the exercises, go through the "deepening by counting" procedure, and then have the client attend to his/her breathing and mentally repeat the word *relax* as he/she exhales. Use the same instructions as before.

5. After the alerting procedure, inquire as to whether the client was able to become deeply relaxed.

6. If there were no problems, have the client begin to use the shorter, 8-muscle-group procedure for home practice.

C. Review and Planning

1. Review the *Weekly Record* and practice record.

2. Instruct client to practice becoming more aware of muscle tension during the day and to try to decrease it.

3. Remind client to continue doing discrimination training during home practice.

4. Remind client of the importance of allowing enough time for complete relaxation between muscle group tension; that is, do not rush through the exercises.

Session 5

A. Session Goals

1. Review records and discuss progress/problems.

2. Repeat 8-muscle-group tension–relaxation procedure.

3. Introduce generalization practice.

B. Session Procedures

1. Repeat 8-muscle-group tension–relaxation training.

2. Encourage the client to begin practicing relaxation in different locations and positions. For example, this week, ask the client to practice relaxation in at least two different rooms. Have the client sit upright during every other practice session, and let the client recline during the alternate practice trials. From this point on, begin varying the client's position while doing in-office relaxation.

C. Review and Planning

1. Review client's progress with relaxation and practice assignments.
2. Review both the *Weekly Record* and the practice records.

Session 6

A. Session Goals

1. Review progress and problems with tension–relaxation practice and any anxiety-provoking situations.
2. Introduce 4-muscle-group tension–relaxation procedure.
3. Assign first homework practice in a low-anxiety situation.

B. Session Procedures

1. Introduce the 4-muscle-group tension–relaxation procedure.
a. Explain that in the session, you will be reducing the number of muscle groups used to 4. This will give the client an even more portable coping strategy.
b. The 4 muscle groups are as follows:
• Both arms
• Chest—"Hold breath, then release"
• Neck—"Slightly hunch shoulders while drawing in and back the neck."
• Face—"Close eyes tightly while drawing up the rest of their face."
c. Complete the tension–relaxation cycles with these 4 groups. Leave at least 30 seconds between tension–relaxation cycles.
d. Go through deepening by counting and attention to breathing exercises as previously described.
2. Instruct the client to practice the 4-muscle-group relaxation technique at least twice a day. Encourage the client to continue to practice in even more different positions and locations. For example, this week, the client could try to practice while standing or walking.
3. Assign the first homework practice in a low-stress situation. The rationale for these *in vivo* homework assignments should be made clear to the client.

We now want to design a homework practice in which you will begin to use your relaxation skills actually to cope with tension and anxiety. The purpose of these assignments is to create opportunities to practice relaxation under controlled conditions—namely, in a situation that you find just a little stressful. Can you think of any events you have scheduled this next week that might be just slightly anxiety-arousing for you?

You and client together should agree on either one mildly stressful situation that occurs repeatedly during the week or two separate mildly stressful events that will occur during the week. We define a low-anxiety situation as a situation that the client scores in the 1–3 range on our 0–8 anxiety rating scale. Make sure that the client will be able to complete at least two *in vivo* practices. For example, practicing relaxation during stressful business meetings or perhaps during hectic parts of the day (e.g., when the children return home from school).

While the situations should be mildly stressful, they should not be so stressful that the client would have difficulty using the relaxation skills successfully. If the client does not easily suggest such events, then suggest that the client create such situations—for example, purposely driving in rush-hour traffic, inviting an unpleasant acquaintance to an activity (e.g., lunch), or volunteering to do some work that is distasteful. The content of the event is perhaps less important than the purpose, which again is to help the client apply the relaxation skills in his/her daily life. The purpose of these practices is not to provide exposure to panic-exciting stimuli but rather to offer a step toward applying the coping strategy. They obviously are early attempts to generalize to *in vivo* situations those skills learned in the office setting.

Clients then receive approved application practices throughout the remainder of the treatment program; after you are confident that the client is able to apply the anxiety-management skills productively in low-stress situations, progressively elevate the homework assignments to more highly stressful situations. For panic clients, the most stressful situations usually are those associated with panic attacks. When some of the anxiety management practices are assigned in panic-associated situations (i.e., in the highest-stress situations), they are, in fact, exposure trials. To this end, these early homework assignments also serve as preparation for *in vivo* exposure. Instruct the client to practice the homework assignment at least two times in the coming week *in addition to* the daily relaxation practice. Instruct the client to record *in vivo* practices on the *Weekly Record* and to mark each of those practices with an asterisk (*).

C. Review and Planning

1. Review progress and problems using the *Weekly Record* and practice records.

Session 7

A. Session Goals

1. Review progress and problems on assigned practice items. Check practice records and *Weekly Record* for accuracy.
2. Repeat 4-muscle-group tension–relaxation exercise.
3. Assign homework practice in a low-stress situation.

B. Session Procedures

1. Repeat 4-muscle-group tension–relaxation procedure.
2. Assign relaxation practice in a place where there is more noise than usual or in situations that have more activity.
3. Assign homework practice in a low-anxiety-producing situation. The client should practice this at least twice in the following week.

C. Review and Planning

1. Review client's progress with relaxation and practice assignments.
2. Review *Weekly Record* and practice records. Make sure to check that the practice assignments were recorded on the bottom half of the *Weekly Record*.

Session 8

A. Session Goals

1. Introduce 4-muscle-group procedure with recall relaxation.
2. Assign home practice in low-anxiety situation.
3. Continue to monitor progress and review records.

B. Session Procedures

1. Introduce relaxation by recall.

a. Explain to the client that one goal of treatment is for him/her to be able to become relaxed readily and quickly.

To help you learn to relax more quickly, I will be asking you to see if you can become relaxed without going through the tension–relaxation cycles. I will ask you to recall what the relaxed state felt like and to try and achieve that state without tensing the muscles.

b. Before starting, arrange for the client to signal you, by raising a forefinger, if he/she has not been able to relax a particular muscle group. Ask client to (1) focus his/her attention on the muscles in his/her hand and arms; (2) very carefully identify any feelings or sensations of tension or tightness that might be present; (3) especially focus on any feelings of tension. (This should be spread over 5 to 10 seconds.)

c. Then (1) ask the client to relax and to recall what it was like when he/she released the tension from that particular muscle group; (2) reemphasize having the client relax, letting go of those particular muscles and allowing them to become more and more deeply relaxed. Allow 30–40 seconds to elapse between interjections of the usual suggestions. Then ask client to signal if the muscles are *not* deeply relaxed. If he/she indicated they are *not* relaxed, try the same suggestions again. If he/she indicated they are *still not* relaxed, then go through the actual tension–relaxation cycle. If he/she indicated they are *relaxed*, go to the next muscle group. Repeat the procedure with the remaining 3 groups.

d. Do not use recall for best tensing; rather use the actual breathing exercise.

e. At the end of relaxation by recall for the 4 muscle groups, again go through (1) the "deepening by counting" and (2) attention to breathing and subvocalizing "relax" with exhalations for about 2 minutes.

2. If the client was *completely* successful with recall, tell him/her to switch to this procedure for home practice. Also, tell him/her that if it does not work at home, he/she should go back to the tension–relaxation cycles and should note on the practice record what difficulties were encountered. This information will help the therapist adjust the relaxation procedure to the individual's needs. In our experience, clients rarely have difficulty learning to do relaxation by recall. Difficulties at this stage of training usually are associated with inadequate practice with the

tension–relaxation exercises; therefore, returning to early training steps usually suffices to remedy the situation.

3. In addition to practicing relaxation by recall, assign a low-anxiety practice. Again, instruct the client to practice this twice before the next session.

4. Also, encourage the client to (a) practice relaxation at work or in other situations where there are more noise and more distractions; (b) continue practice in different positions.

C. Review and Planning

1. Note progress in therapy and the status of the client's records.
2. Note time and date of next appointment.

Session 9

A. Session Goals

1. Repeat 4-muscle-group recall.
2. Assign home practice in moderate-anxiety situations.
3. Review progress/problems, and check records.

B. Session Procedures

1. Repeat 4-muscle-group recall procedure as listed in previous session.
2. Assign home practice in moderate-anxiety situation. Remind the client to practice the assignment at least twice before the next session.
3. Encourage the client to continue relaxation practice in different positions and situations.

C. Review and Planning

1. Review client's progress with relaxation and practice assignments.
2. Make sure practice assignments are correctly recorded on the *Weekly Record*.

D. Progress Note

1. Note progress, therapy, and the status of the client's records.
2. Note time and date of next appointment.

Session 10

A. Session Goals

1. Review progress and problems on assigned practice items.
2. Introduce and practice cue-controlled relaxation.
3. Assign continued moderate-anxiety practice.

B. Session Procedures

1. Introduce cue-controlled relaxation. Before leaving this step, make sure the client fully understands the cue-controlled procedure, the rationale for the procedure, and how to use the procedure as a coping strategy. Practice the procedure *at least* twice during the session.

With this procedure, the client will have a readily portable coping strategy. The client should be encouraged to use cue-controlled relaxation during the day whenever he/she begins to feel tension. By this training session, the client should be able to identify easily low levels of tension in muscles that should be relaxed. If clients are having difficulty monitoring low tension levels, then we suggest repeating the discrimination training exercises. We usually apply these exercises to the muscle groups the client has most difficulty with.

To begin cue-controlled relaxation, have the client focus on his/her breathing, then take a deep breath and think the word "relax." Repeat this procedure several times, and pair the word "relax" with exhalation. Thinking the word "relax" then becomes a cue for relaxation. The purpose of cue-controlled relaxation is to provide the client with a highly portable and effective means of dealing with tension and anxiety when the tension is still at a low level. It also increases the client's confidence that he/she can control anxiety levels. In this way, the client is using the procedure to cope with the beginning of tension and anxiety. The client should try to use the cue-controlled procedure several times daily. Encourage the client to practice these relaxation procedures at every possible opportunity and again in different locations and/or body positions.

2. Assign a moderately anxiety-provoking homework assignment, and record the assignment in the progress note.

3. Explain to the client that he/she is to continue recording any use of the relaxation procedures even though he/she may be using them more frequently now.

C. Review and Planning

Review progress and problems using the *Weekly Record* and practice records.

Session 11

A. Session Goals

1. Review progress and problems.
2. Repeat cue-controlled relaxation.
3. Assign home practice in a high-anxiety situation.

B. Session Procedures

1. Repeat cue-controlled relaxation as described in the previous session. Have the client practice this procedure twice during the session.

2. Encourage the client to practice cue-controlled relaxation whenever he/she begins to notice tension. Make sure the client practices this procedure at work, at home, and in other situations.

3. Assign home practice in a high-anxiety situation. A high-anxiety situation falls in the 6–8 range on our 0–8 anxiety scale. By this session, the relaxation practices should be taking place in situations associated with panic attacks and/or applied during *in vivo* exposures to panic symptoms.

C. Review and Planning

1. Review progress and problems.
2. Check accuracy of *Weekly Record* and practice records.

Sessions 12, 13, and 14

A. Session Goals

1. Review progress and problems.
2. Devote this time to enhancing the generalization of the client's skills to any additional areas that have not been covered in practice assignments previously.
3. Assign home practice in high-anxiety situations.

B. Session Procedures

1. Discuss additional areas where the client needs to practice using his/her relaxation skills. The goal here is to facilitate generalization of the strategy for coping with anxiety. Generalization and maintenance of treatment effects may be facilitated in several ways. First, ask the client to prepare a list of activities and situations that are likely to occur over the next few months and in which they will practice their newly learned skills. Encourage the client to include in this list a few recurring activities (e.g., going shopping, as well as more novel situations such as attending a seasonal event or celebrating a birthday). Explain that the client is to examine the list regularly and to add to it or delete items from it as their life situation changes. The client is to use this list to help reward him/herself to continue to practice anxiety management skills. Second, re-emphasize the need to continue to expose him/herself to panic-associated situations and to activities that induce panic-like symptoms and to use the relaxation skills in those situations. Third, forewarn the client that he/she may occasionally have a panic attack. Encourage the client to see those occasional attacks as opportunities to retrain in the therapeutic procedures.

Because what they have learned in therapy is a set of skills, those skills will become "rusty" if not employed on a regular basis. In fact, the recurrence of panic symptoms may signal that the therapeutic skills are not being well maintained or used. Also encourage clients to share the newly learned skills with spouses, children, and close friends because teaching others how to use relaxation is a good way to solidify the skills. In addition, family members may then help with maintenance of treatment gains by encouraging the client to use the skills in stressful situations. Essentially, any strategy that increases the likelihood of the client routinely practicing relaxation skills and exposing him/herself to stressful situations will facilitate generalizations of treatment effects. The better you tailor generalization procedures to the client's life situation, the better will be the results. The use of generalization procedures will lead to a good long-term treatment outcome.

2. Assign home practice in areas identified in Item 1 above as well as a high-anxiety situation. Each of these exercises should be practiced at least twice.

C. Review and Planning

1. Review the client's progress in relaxation in different situations on the *Weekly Record* and practice records.

2. Check for accuracy on the records.

Session 15: Generalization Practice and Termination Issues

A. Session Goals

1. Review progress in treatment.

2. Remind the client to continue practicing relaxation on a daily basis.

3. Review treatment progress and give instructions for the next (6) months.

4. Schedule posttreatment assessments.

B. Session Procedures

1. Inquire as to client's general status as well as success with homework assignments. Check the practice monitoring sheets.

2. Review the *Weekly Record* for accuracy as well as for signs of specific problems that have developed for the client.

3. Practice cue-controlled relaxation at least twice during the session. Assess the client's facility with cue-controlled relaxation.

4. Tell the client to begin to use cue-controlled relaxation as an active coping strategy whenever he/she becomes aware of any tension. The client should practice cue-controlled relaxation regularly throughout the day in as many different situations as possible in order to maximize generalization.

5. Verbally review all of the relaxation procedures and the accompanying rationale with the client, including:

   a. 16-muscle groups

   b. 8-muscle groups

   c. 4-muscle groups

   d. Discrimination training

   e. Recall relaxation

   f. Cue-controlled relaxation

   g. Use of relaxation as a coping strategy and the need to practice

   h. Evaluation and recording of the client's progress and facility with each of these techniques

6. Because this is the client's last therapy session, do a general review of the client's progress in treatment and attend to termination issues. Instruct the client to continue to use the coping strategies he/she has learned during treatment, and encourage the client to continue to assign homework activities for him/herself. Remind the client that the clinic will contact the client for 6- and 12-month follow-ups, but if the client has questions about therapy progress or procedures or runs into a situation with which it is difficult to cope, he/she should feel free to telephone the clinic. Also, mention that if necessary, the clinic is, of course, available for crisis intervention. Schedule the client for posttreatment assessment, and remind the client about formal 6- and 12-month follow-ups.

7. Complete the posttreatment assessment.

C. Review and Planning

Spend some time dealing with any unresolved termination issues and solidifying rapport with the client. Encourage the client again to practice daily the coping strategies he/she has learned in as many different situations as possible, in order to maximize generalization. Remind the client again about follow-up assessments.

Check to make sure all of the necessary data have been collected and that the client's needs have been met as well as possible within the framework of this protocol. Remind the client that continued practice is necessary to maintain gains and continue improvements.

6

Cognitive Treatment Component

The cognitive therapy component of our panic treatment protocol is adapted from the Beck and Emery (1979) treatment protocol for anxiety disorders; this cognitive treatment manual has now been elaborated into a book that we highly recommend (Beck & Emery, 1985). Our application of Beck and Emery's techniques is based on a skills training approach in which patients learn a variety of cognitive skills for coping with stress and anxiety and for reevaluating their beliefs about and appraisal of both environmental and internal (physiological) cues. In addition, clients practice applying these coping strategies both during therapy sessions and in homework assignments between sessions.

While the cognitive component of our treatment protocol follows a structured format, it also demands considerably more flexibility than do the other two components in our treatment protocol. The cognitive component requires more direct verbal interaction with the clients than does either the relaxation or the exposure component of the treatment protocol. In order to use the cognitive therapy component of this treatment protocol effectively, the therapist should be experienced in the application of Beck and Emery's cognitive approach. Because of the complexity of the cognitive treatment, therapists usually find the cognitive component of the panic treatment protocol the most challenging to apply and the most difficult to teach their clients.

In our clinical setting, we find that continual review and training in the application of the cognitive component to panic clients is both helpful and perhaps even necessary to maintain the level of skill that allows facility with the technique. In addition to weekly staffings in which case progress is reviewed and treatment techniques are discussed, we also use role playing of the treatment procedures as well as the study of videotape and audiotape sessions of actual cognitive treatment sessions. We find that these procedures help maintain the skill level necessary to execute the cognitive component of the panic treatment protocol with clarity and facility.

The initial phase of the cognitive therapy component provides an introduction to cognitive therapy as well as basic education in the premises of cognitive coping strategies. During this introductory phase, as elaborated in "Session 2," the client basically receives didactic instruction. This initial phase is then followed by a second phase (several sessions) during which the client learns a variety of cognitive strategies for coping with stress, anxiety, and panic attacks. During the final and longest phase of the cognitive component, the client is instructed in the application and practice of these cognitive coping strategies. It is in this third phase that the client practices applying the cognitive coping strategies learned in earlier therapy sessions both during and between therapy sessions. Therefore, during this third phase of the cognitive component we emphasize our conceptualization of cognitive therapy as a process in which the client learns and practices a variety of coping skills. These cognitive skills are designed to improve the client's ability to manage stress and to cope with anxiety reactions and symptoms regarding panic attacks. The cognitive techniques are integrated with the exposure procedures.

The remainder of this chapter presents a detailed session-by-session protocol for the presentation of the cognitive therapy treatment component. The format is the same as the relaxation protocol (i.e., starting with the second session; the first session, "treatment explanation," is presented in Chapter 4). As in Chapter 5, the goals, procedures, and planning strategy cues are provided for each session. We have included verbatim illustrations throughout the protocol in order to make clearer the *content* of the procedure. These examples should not be seen as scripts to be read or memorized and presented to the client. Rather, the therapist should translate the procedure into a comfortable personal style and tailor the content to the client's specific needs. We also remind the reader that while we have presented each of the three major components of the panic treatment manual separately, in actual practice, all three components are presented to the patient in an integrated fashion. Accordingly, the treatment rationale already should have been discussed with the client during the first therapy session. Because the first four therapy sessions are devoted largely to progressive relaxation training, proportionately less time is devoted to cognitive therapy in these early sessions. For the most part, the first four cognitive therapy sessions are devoted to didactic presentation of the foundation skills for monitoring cognitions and comprehending the foundation procedures for the cognitive coping strategies.

As therapy progresses, proportionately more time is devoted to cognitive therapy techniques. The schedule of sessions for the cognitive component was presented in Chapter 4, Table 4-1.

Session 2

A. Session Goals

1. Discuss episodes of heightened anxiety that have occurred since the previous session.
2. Begin to identify antecedents to the anxiety.
3. Introduce techniques for monitoring cognitions and self-statements.

B. Session Procedures

1. Review the *Weekly Record* with the client. Discuss any episodes of heightened anxiety, and begin to have the client try to identify any specific antecedents to anxiety. Inquire as to how the client dealt with these situations. Tell the client that he/she will learn to become more aware of tension/anxiety at earlier stages and will learn to respond differently to these situations.

2. Introduce cognitive monitoring. Maladaptive cognitions have two major characteristics: (a) they are automatic; and (b) they are very discrete predictions or interpretations of a given situation. The term *automatic* means that these cognitions often occur very rapidly in certain situations and may be outside of the person's awareness. The term *discrete* refers to the fact that these cognitions are often very specific in content and include very specific interpretations and predictions about the situation. The implication for treatment is that the client must first learn to become more clearly aware of the kinds of self-statements that he/she is making in anxiety-provoking situations, and that he/she must learn to pursue the thought until he/she arrives at the very specific content or prediction that is contributing to the increased anxiety.

During the sessions, you can serve as a model and coach for this kind of self-monitoring and critical analysis of anxiety-provoking thoughts. For example, a client may say, "I am afraid of having a panic attack during our weekly business meeting." In responding to such a statement, you should ask questions that are designed to elicit specific interpretations and predictions being made by the client in the situation—for example, "What do you think will happen?" or "What do you picture happening?" or "What are you telling yourself about the situation?" In response to these questions, the client may produce more specific statements such as, "I am afraid that other people will notice I'm nervous, that I won't be able to talk, and that I will look like a fool." Statements such as these can provide the material that the therapist and client will work with during the therapy sessions.

Cognitive monitoring should be introduced with the following statements:

Now let's take a look at one situation in your life that is anxiety provoking for you and try to look at the thoughts you're having in that situation. As you practice thought monitoring over the next few weeks, you will be able to reevaluate your anxiety-provoking thoughts.

Explain that the first step in learning to deal with worrisome thoughts is to become aware of which cognitions are anxiety producing for the client. To this end, the client will attempt to monitor anxiety-arousing cognitions and self-statements during the next week. The client should record the cognitions, if possible, on the *Weekly Record* (see Appendix A). These recorded cognitions will be used in future therapy sessions in order to develop cognitive coping strategies. Follow a general sequence of questioning that will facilitate uncovering the very specific predictions and interpretations that the client is making with questions such as, "What are you saying to yourself in this situation?" and "What do you imagine will happen in this situation?" If the client makes a very general statement, try to elicit more specific predictions and interpretations by simply asking, "Then what?" Once a specific prediction or interpretation has been elicited from the client, proceed to show the client how to record the thought or self-statement on the monitoring sheet. In future sessions, use these data in the logical analysis of the client's automatic thoughts. In order to assure that the client has a good grasp of the procedure, you may want to request a return demonstration.

C. Review and Planning

1. Briefly review and summarize the material presented in this session.

2. Review the importance of recording automatic thoughts on the *Weekly Record.*

3. Review the procedures for cognitive monitoring.

Session 3

A. Session Goals

1. Review client record sheets, and discuss progress/problems.
2. Emphasize importance of noticing tension early on, so the client can begin to cope with the anxiety/tension at an earlier stage.
3. Present didactic material on exploring alternative explanations for cognitive self-statements.

B. Session Procedures

1. Review the client's *Weekly Record*, checking that the cognitive monitoring and data collection was completed accurately. Fill in any gaps in the data. Remind the client that it takes time to practice and learn these procedures and that it may be several weeks before the client feels confident with the cognitive material. The last point is especially important if the client is discouraged.

2. During this session, introduce the technique of exploring alternative explanations while reviewing the client's cognitive monitoring data from the *Weekly Record*. Do not dwell on the concept of alternative explanations too long, but make sure that the client understands the concept. When possible, the client should begin to list alternatives for stressful situations on the *Weekly Record*.

The concept of exploring alternatives can be presented in the following way:

Very often, people have a narrow or limited view of anxiety-provoking situations because they usually focus on the worst possible interpretations or outcomes. The first step in changing your thoughts about a situation is to ask yourself whether or not there are alternative ways of looking at the situation.

For example, if you notice that your boss or your spouse seems angry, you may think, "He/she must be upset with me; I must have done something wrong." When you find yourself jumping to this conclusion, you could ask yourself whether there are other reasons for the person's behavior. Alternative explanations might be that the person is cranky because of pressure from work situations, or that he/she is angry at someone else, or that this person behaves this way almost all the time regardless of what you do.

In other situations, you may be saying to yourself things like, "I know I am going to fail," or "I know I am going to be very anxious in this situation." When you find yourself making such predictions or interpretations in a situation, you should treat these statements as guesses or hypotheses rather than as facts, and ask yourself, "How do I know that this will happen?" or "What evidence do I have that this will happen?" or "Are there other equally likely ways of looking at the situation?"

At this point, some clients may become skeptical and ask something like, "Are you telling me that I'm always wrong about situations?" or "Are you saying that all I have to do is look on the bright side of things?" One way to respond to this type of question might be as follows:

No, we recognize that some situations and some people are objectively difficult and hard to deal with. What we are saying here is that you may be focusing too much on the negative aspects of the situations, and because of this negative focus you may be incorrectly jumping to anxiety-provoking conclusions. What I am suggesting here is that you begin to consider other ways of looking at anxiety-provoking situations and focus on ways to solve the problems you face.

At this point, it may be helpful to demonstrate the utility of this approach by asking the client to provide an example from his/her own life. For example, "Can you think of any times recently when you caught yourself jumping to a negative conclusion that created anxiety and that you later found out was an incorrect interpretation or an incorrect prediction?" Most clients will be able to provide some kind of example. If not, suggest some possibilities based on the cognitive monitoring data or from information contained in the client's clinical record.

One rather common cognition for panic patients is that a noticeable change in their physical status is the beginning of a panic attack. Predictions that panic attacks will lead to heart attacks, loss of control, or even death are not uncommon. Similarly, predictions that entering either specific situations associated with panic or generally stressful situations will lead to a panic attack seem instrumentally related to anticipatory anxiety. For all of these cognitions, encourage the client to search for alternative explanations. In any case, explain that a large part of the work done in the therapy sessions and at home will be to learn how to identify and isolate these anxiety-provoking thoughts.

C. Progress Note

1. Note progress in therapy, how the didactic presentation went, and any other relevant observations.
2. Note next appointment date and time.

Session 4

A. Session Goals

1. Review records and discuss progress/problems. Assess the client's understanding and use of exploration of alternative explanations presented during the previous session.
2. Introduce analysis of faulty logic.

B. Session Procedures

1. Introduction to cognitively evaluating faulty logic

Therapist Reminder. Following are some general guidelines for the types of questions to use during the analysis of faulty logic. However, the general format for this procedure should be to remind the client that he/she is now treating his/her thoughts as hypotheses or guesses rather than facts, and that he/she should examine the evidence for his/her predictions. Do not simply tell the client that he/she has made a particular type of error, but instead ask the client to examine the contents of his/her statements, and then try to decide whether or not he/she has made one of the particular logical errors.

In the course of such questioning, the client may bring up other predictions or interpretations that also may be subjected to the analysis of faulty logic. You may decide either to pursue these additional predictions immediately or to make a note of them for discussion at future sessions; however, the best strategy is to return periodically to the original prediction or interpretation under discussion and to ask the client if he/she is now able to reevaluate the cognition in some way. With enough discussion, most clients will usually acknowledge at least a small change in their degree of belief in a prediction or interpretation. Very often, the predictions or interpretations a client makes are catastrophic and highly unlikely to occur. The following section includes various types of client predictions and interpretations, and possible therapist responses during the analysis of faulty logic or decatastrophizing phases.

Simple declarative statements from the client can often be challenged by asking how the client knows that this is the case or where the evidence is that this is true—for example:

> CLIENT: My boss was grouchy today, he must not have liked the report that I turned in last week.

THERAPIST: How do you know that his anger was directed at you? [or] Did he actually say anything to you to make you think that he was unhappy with your report?

CLIENT: I really made a fool of myself at the staff meeting.
THERAPIST: How do you know that?
CLIENT: I really had a big panic attack!
THERAPIST: Well, you may have had a panic attack, but what makes you say that you did badly? Are you sure that anybody really noticed?

There may be times during the discussion when the client produces absolutistic, overgeneralized statements such as, "I am a failure," or "I am a poor mother," or "I can't handle anxiety." Respond to such statements similarly to the following:

There may be times when you don't do as well as you like, but are there other times when you do perform satisfactorily?

After some discussion, the client will usually acknowledge at least a few instances in which his/her performance was adequate. You can then ask:

Then isn't it a kind of overgeneralization to call yourself a failure [poor mother, incompetent worker, etc.]?

Very often, questions and comments by the client regarding the therapy or the therapist may be a source of material for analysis of faulty logic. The general strategy here is to ask what thoughts prompted the comment or question. Comments such as,

You probably think I am a real basket case? or Do you think that this therapy will really work for me?

can be dealt with in the following manner:

Well, let's see if we can get at some of the thoughts that you are having about this. What are you saying to yourself right now?

Such an inquiry will usually yield a number of overgeneralized catastrophic types of statements that can then be subjected to critical analysis.

2. Faulty logic: Explanation to the client

As I have already explained, anxiety in certain situations may be exacerbated by your interpretations or what you say to yourself in those situations. In the next two sessions, we will look at some techniques to change your negative self-statements by questioning and challenging your interpretations and assumptions. Using some of the entries from your self-monitoring sheets, I'll show you how you can learn to challenge your negative thoughts by asking yourself questions about how you arrived at the conclusion that increased anxiety. As you learn these techniques, you will be able to cope with anxiety by asking yourself similar questions when you find yourself feeling anxious outside of therapy.

The basic idea here is to ask yourself (a) how you are interpreting certain situations and (b) some of the negative predictions that you are making. These kinds of self-statements often precipitate anxiety. Once you isolate these predictions, you'll learn to treat them as beliefs or hypotheses rather than as facts. The general strategy is to begin to question and to challenge these hypotheses by examining the evidence for them and examining how you arrived at your conclusions.

Achieving control of your anxiety is a learned skill, somewhat like learning to ride a bicycle. To be really effective, you must practice regularly. Also, as you practice, you should begin to be more aware of the tension you experience to be able to recognize it earlier, and to deal with it so that it becomes something with which you can more readily cope.

For this training to be of the most benefit to you, you should practice the exercises at least twice per day. If you cannot find time for two practices per day, one is acceptable but not as good as twice per day. If you cannot, or will not, practice regularly, then you probably will not receive the major benefits of this training.

3. Faulty logic: Introduction to evaluating logical errors. Introduce the client to the various types of errors that lead to faulty logic. After a brief introduction to error types and the analysis of faulty logic, name each of the errors and give a general example. Then invite the client to generate examples of the error from instances in his/her own life. The client should be able to produce at least one or two examples, and these may serve as material for the work in later sessions.

The discussion of logical errors can be introduced in the following manner:

We have found that people make certain kinds of errors in the way they look at situations, and that these errors in thinking contribute to arriving at incorrect, anxiety-provoking predictions and conclusions. I'm going to describe briefly some of the major kinds of errors and give you an example of each of them; then perhaps you can give me an example from your own life. At first, it is not unusual to have difficulty coming up with an example because, as we said before, many of these conclusions are "automatic" and can occur without you even noticing them. Of course, after we discuss these errors in the next sessions, you will be better able to catch yourself making these errors in your everyday life. And, of course, being able to catch yourself making these errors is the first step toward being able to change them.

a. Evidence

The most general error, of course, is jumping to a conclusion before you consider all of the facts or all of the evidence. For example, you may assume that you are going to fail a test or do poorly on a task, overlooking the fact that you have prepared very carefully for the exam or that you have successfully completed the same or similar tasks on other occasions. Or, a friend, spouse, or boss may be acting in a hostile or cold manner and you automatically assume that they are displeased with you, overlooking other factors that may be contributing to how they are acting, such as, being in a bad mood, being angry at someone else, etcetera.

b. Overgeneralizing

We often make negative predictions or conclusions about a situation, based on a very limited set of past examples. For example, you may predict that you will fail an exam or become very anxious in a certain situation because you have done poorly on similar exams or have been anxious in similar situations in the past. You may be overlooking several instances in which you did well on such exams or were not anxious in such situations. Whenever you find yourself making a negative prediction about your ability to handle some future situation, you should ask yourself, "Have I had only failures in this situation in the past, or have there actually been times when I did okay?"

c. Certainties versus possibilities

In many situations, especially those that are anxiety provoking, we tend to confuse low probabilities with high probabilities or to act and feel as though negative outcomes are certainties rather than possibilities. For example, the following statements may be realistic: "I could do poorly on this exam"; "I may get into a fight with my boss." Unrealistic statements that turn possibilities into certainties are statements such as "I know I am going to panic next time I have to make a speech"; or "I know that my boss is going to be angry with me." When you notice yourself making such unrealistic statements, you should ask yourself "What are the real odds of this happening?"

4. All-or-none thinking

We often think in black-or-white, all-or-none terms instead of recognizing that almost nothing is either/or and that there are gradations or degrees of anxiety, skill, and good or bad performances. Many perfectionists implicitly believe that they must do a job perfectly or they have failed completely. In such situations, the person mistakenly equates one mistake with total failure.

5. Absolutistic thinking

In anxiety-provoking situations, we often think in absolute terms, or we give ourselves ultimatums. You should be alert to statements that include words such as "always," "never," "need," "must," "can't," and be alert to overgeneralized labels such as "I am a failure" or "I am an incompetent worker" or "I am a bad mother, father, husband, wife," and so on. You can begin to learn to replace the *absolute* type of words with more *relative* terms. For example, "always" can be replaced with "often." "Never" can be replaced by "rarely." The phrase, "I need," "I have to," "I must" can be replaced by phrases such as "I prefer," "I want to," and so on. The phrase "I can't" can be replaced with the phrase "I would find it difficult."

In further discussion of these errors, take care to label the error for the client and to ask the client to be on the lookout for that type of error during the course of the next week. As therapy progresses and as the client becomes more efficient at identifying the errors, encourage the client to identify and label the error.

C. Review and Planning

1. Review the *Weekly Records* and practice records.
2. Remind the client to begin to identify logical errors in thinking.
3. Review the procedures for cognitive monitoring and remedy and problems.

Session 5

A. Session Goals

1. Review records and discuss progress/problems in monitoring automatic thoughts.

2. Present didactic instruction for:
a. Decatastrophizing
b. Rescue factors
c. Reattribution
d. Hypothesis testing—behavioral experiments
3. Consider using a handout on logical errors and methods of dealing with them to review the didactic presentation.

Therapist Reminder

1. Review the client's progress and accuracy in self-monitoring of anxiety and automatic thoughts. Emphasize the importance of keeping accurate records because these records will provide important material for therapy. Reinforce the client for accurate and consistent self-monitoring. Spend 10–15 minutes at the beginning of *each* session reviewing the client's previous week. Avoid reviewing everything that happened during the previous week; rather, focus on reviewing the outcome of homework assignments and dealing with problems regarding treatment progress.

2. Present the didactic instruction on decatastrophizing and then discuss the use of rescue factors and hypothesis testing as coping tactics. Try to draw on the client's idiosyncratic situations from the list of automatic thoughts in order to exemplify the instructional material for the client.

B. Session Procedures

1. Present the following didactic material.
a. Decatastrophizing. In addition to the specific techniques that are included in the analysis of faulty logic, a second major technique is that of *decatastrophizing or "what if."* This technique is usually used after a detailed analysis of faulty logic. After you and the client have subjected the client's predictions or interpretations to analysis of faulty logic, the client may acknowledge that his/her negative or catastrophic prediction is probably not as likely as he/she originally thought. You can support the client's reinterpretation of the situation, but then go one step further by asking, "Let's assume for the moment that the worst possible thing actually happened. What would be the result of it happening?" Decatastrophizing or "what if" can be introduced after the discussion of logical errors in the following way?

We have just looked at some ways that you can arrive at a more realistic interpretation and fewer negative predictions about certain situations, but sometimes it can be helpful to ask yourself,"What if the worst were actually to come true?" For example, if you're worried about failing a test or having an argument with your boss, you may be able to find errors in your thinking that permit you to reevaluate this possibility. However, at that point, it may be helpful to shift gears in your thinking and ask yourself, "Well, what if the worst possible thing were to come true?" "What if I did have a panic attack or what if I did faint?" Your first reaction to this question is probably something like, "That would be awful or terrible," or "My life, would be in jeopardy," etcetera. However, you may find that when you think carefully and critically about these assumptions, and subject them to analysis of errors, that you have prematurely jumped to negative conclusions.

For example, when you think about the consequences of a panic attack you may automatically say to yourself, "If I panic while driving home from work, I'd cause an accident and kill someone or die myself." When you make this prediction explicit, and then subject it to logical analysis, you may find that you have made some sort of error such as overgeneralizing from a limited set of examples, overlooking other evidence, etcetera.

In the preceding example, the client should logically review the probability of having a panic attack in that situation; his/her driving history; the likelihood of being completely incapacitated during a panic attack; and so on. Similarly, when you think about the consequences of stumbling over your words while making a presentation to your colleagues, you may automatically think they will think, "I'm a fool" and not even consider alternative possibilities, such as they will not even notice you stumbling over your words; or even if they do notice, no one will really care. You can even take this one step further and ask yourself, "Well, what if some of the people in the audience do think that I look foolish, does it really matter what these people think?" As you begin focusing in on these thoughts, you will probably experience an increase in anxiety because the thoughts themselves are anxiety-provoking. However, you should keep on with the logical analysis of your thoughts, and through this process, the thoughts themselves will become less anxiety-provoking, and easier to change.

The general strategy for decatastrophizing is to encourage the client to outline specifically the consequences of the feared event. By now, the client's specific prediction has already been subjected to analysis of faulty logic. But at some point, shift the focus of discussion, and ask the client to think more precisely about what would happen if his/her worst fear were actually to come true. In the case of a panic patient, ask questions such as, "What would happen if other people noticed how anxious you were?" or "Suppose you did faint while talking with your boss?" For the client who is concerned about avoiding or escaping from panic-provoking situations, questions might be, "What would happen if you suddenly left your office?" or "What if you could not possibly leave the situation?"

One immediate effect of these kinds of questions is that the client's anxiety level increases. At this point, you might say,

I know that it's difficult to think about this situation, but if we follow the logic of the situation, I think you'll find that the anxiety subsides somewhat.

Once the client has discussed some of the expected consequences of the feared event, he/she and you are better able to evaluate whether in fact these consequences would be as intolerable as the client believes they would be or whether the client's anxiety or embarrassment would be time-limited. Very often, the feared event has global and overgeneralized implications for the client's evaluation of him/herself. For example, a client may report, "If I have a panic attack, I won't be able to do my work and I'll get fired," or "If I have panic attacks, it means that I have no control over my life." Should such cognitions be uncovered, use the techniques described in the analysis of faulty logic to help the client recognize that such conclusions are unwarranted generalizations.

b. Rescue factors. A detailed discussion of feared consequences also permits exploration of measures that can be taken to correct the situation. For example, the client who fears making mistakes on a new job may not have considered the possibility that his/her supervisor might recognize that this is a normal part of the breaking-in process and would be willing to answer questions and offer assistance if the client simply asks. Many panic clients fear being totally incapacitated by panic and as a result find themselves in jeopardy, fearing that a panic-induced heart attack could be fatal. Such clients have not considered rescue factors such as persons in the situation that would be helpful; the various and successful treatments for cardiac conditions; the availability of ambulance service; proximity of a hospital; and so on. Because she/he has avoided thinking the situation through, the client may have overlooked many of these straightforward *rescue factors*; and a consideration of these factors may put the feared event into a more realistic, less catastrophic perspective.

c. Hypothesis testing. This technique is also designed to encourage the client to monitor negative cognitions and to make more realistic predictions about feared events. Hypothesis testing involves a series of behavioral experiments in which the client writes out catastrophic predictions about various situations he/she is likely to encounter during the week. During subsequent sessions, the client and you can examine the evidence that either supports or refutes these predictions. In this manner, the client can experience directly that few, if any, or his/her dire predictions come true. Have the client keep a record of the dire predictions that he/she makes during the week and the actual consequences of the event that led to the prediction. Using these data, the client and you can evaluate both the frequency and the accuracy of the predictions.

Many panic clients make catastrophic predictions about the effects of anxiety on their ability to function. A client might say, "I am too anxious to read," or "I am too anxious to make a phone call." If the client is experiencing anxiety in the session, predictions such as these can be tested during the session by actually having the client attempt these activities. Beck and Emery (1979) call these activities behavioral experiments. On completing such an experiment, many clients may protest that they "did not do very well," but you can point out that even though performance may not have been perfect, the client was able to do it, contrary to the prediction. Of course, do not attempt such an experiment until you have some idea of the kinds of activities that the client *can* carry out successfully.

Evaluate other catastrophic predictions such as, "I wouldn't be able to drive during a panic atack," or "If I have a bad anxiety attack while I'm at home alone with my baby, I won't be able to care for him" on the basis of the client's *Weekly Record.* Very often these records contain clear evidence that, in fact, the client can drive, care for children, and carry out a number of activities while experiencing rather severe anxiety. As therapy progresses and the client learns to cope with anxiety more effectively, additional examples of how inaccurate and catastrophic predictions govern the panic patient's behavior.

d. Reattribution. In addition to facilitating analysis of faulty logic, at some time during this session, introduce the technique of reattribution. This technique is intended to enhance the effectiveness of the other cognitive techniques and to serve as additional tools the client can use to reevaluate his/her thoughts. This is a specific cognitive technique focused on a common tendency among anxious clients to assume total responsibility for a given event and to worry about possible future events over which they have no control.

For example, if a man has a first date with a woman who proves to be cold and disinterested, he might automatically assume responsibility for her behavior because he feels he is boring or unattractive. He may overlook other factors such as illness or fatigue, or that this woman may have a cold or hold a disinterested attitude toward most of her dates. In all instances, directly ask the client, "How much responsibility do you really have for _____?" or conversely, "Could there be other reasons for _____?" In the preceding example, you might also ask, "How do you know that she was disinterested because she found you boring or unattractive?" and "Is it possible that there are other reasons for the way she behaved which have nothing to do with you?"

In any situation in which the client appears to be assuming the responsibility for a particular problem, attempt to sort out those aspects of the problem over which the client realistically has little or no control. This will have the dual effect of relieving the client of the unrealistic burden of self-imposed responsibility and help bring into clearer focus those aspects of the situation that the client may actually be able to change. As can be seen from the example, helping the client to reattribute the responsibility of certain events involves the use of other cognitive techniques, such as exploration of alternatives and examining the evidence.

2. If desired, give the client a handout summarizing instructional components from the previous two cognitive therapy sessions.

C. Review and Planning

1. Give the client new *Weekly Record* sheets, and reemphasize the need to keep consistent and accurate records, including automatic thoughts and anxiety-arousing situations. Remind the client that self-monitoring is an important skill that needs to be practiced and that this procedure is an important part of the treatment program.

2. Instruct the client to start to note on the *Weekly Records* automatic thoughts and thinking errors that the client finds him/herself making.

3. Explain that during the next session, more time will be focused on applying the cognitive coping strategies discussed in this session.

Session 6

A. Session Goals

1. Review progress and difficulties with cognitive monitoring and with previously presented didactic material, and subject any anxiety-provoking situations to logical analysis.

2. Assign first homework practice.

Therapist Reminder

1. During this phase of treatment, the client will practice the application of the various coping strategies that have been introduced in earlier

sessions. Each of the remaining sessions will involve three parts: (a) review of progress and problems during the past week, with a special emphasis on the use of cognitive coping strategies during homework assignments; (b) covert rehearsal of cognitive coping strategies during graduated imaginal exposure; (c) development and assignment of individualized behavioral experiments associated with *in vivo* homework assignments, which are to be completed before the next treatment session.

2. Review the client's progress and any problems related to homework or data collection during the previous week. Spend 10–15 minutes at the beginning of each of the remaining sessions reviewing the client's past week. Avoid a review of everything that happened during the week. Focus on any problems or progress and on reviewing the outcome of behavioral experiments and suggestions.

3. Adopt a problem-solving approach to dealing with the client's problems. Encourage the client to adopt the same type of approach by asking him/herself the questions: "What was the situation? What happened? How did the client attempt to deal with the situation? Did the client try to employ coping strategies learned during treatment? If not, why not? If coping strategies were used, what seemed to be the difficulty with them? How could the strategies be applied differently? What can be learned from this problem or experience?" Try to avoid a completely negative view of the situation. It is not unusual for the client at this stage of therapy to have difficulty completing assignments. As is typical of thinking patterns, the client may tend to catastrophize these difficulties and to label the situation as "total failures." Once again, logically analyze that interpretation and try to identify some positive or educational aspects of the problem or situation.

4. Show the client how to record problematic thoughts and which cognitive coping strategies are to be used during the next week.

B. Session Procedures

1. Review the client's *Weekly Record*, attending carefully to the list of automatic thoughts and errors in thinking. By this time, the client should demonstrate a clear understanding of thinking errors and be able to identify such errors on the self-monitoring records. Therapy should not proceed until you are sure the client is able to grasp well these fundamental skills (i.e., self-monitoring and basic comprehension of thinking errors). At this point in treatment, clients do not have to be proficient in the application of these cognitive tactics to anxiety situations; however, the client should have a solid understanding of the

rationale and basic content of cognitive behavior therapy. If such is not the case, review and discuss further the didactic material presented in earlier sessions. Either role-played or other *in vivo* practices may be helpful.

2. Application of coping strategies during graded visualizations of anxiety-eliciting stimuli. In the sixth treatment session, begin to prepare the client for both imaginal and *in vivo* exposure therapy by providing training in imagery visualization and easily accomplished homework practices. At the same time, use these opportunities to encourge the clients to practice cognitive coping strategies. Explain to the client that the practice of the cognitive skills is an ongoing and necessary activity. While it may be difficult to arrange real-life practice situations, it is quite easy to imagine such situations and at least in imagination to see oneself using the cognitive strategies. Such practice allows the client to plan which cognitive skills will be most useful for certain situations and how to employ these specific skills. Mention that the cognitive techniques are ways to manage panic and anxiety in stressful situations, but the core treatment for panic disorder is the exposure therapy. In the following treatment sessions, the client will be exposing him/herself to panic-provoking situations and anxiety-eliciting stimuli both in imagination and in real life. The invocation of the cognitive coping strategies in these exposure trials serves two purposes: (a) to help the client enter and remain actively engaged in the scene or situation and (b) to provide practice with the cognitive management techniques. Thus, over the next several sessions, the client will practice the cognitive management techniques both covertly during visualization of stressful scenes and *in vivo* during assigned homework. The specific procedure for developing the graduated panic hierarchy, visualization practices, and *in vivo* assignments are presented in Chapter 7.

3. Introduce cognitive coping practice. Assign the first cognitive homework practice in a low-anxiety situation. Toward the end of each session, during the application practice phase of treatment, you and the client should collaborate to develop one or more specific homework assignments. These homework assignments can be conceptualized as "behavioral experiments," designed to test the validity of the client's beliefs about anxiety and stress and to practice coping with interfering thoughts. These behavioral experiments will be assigned for homework between sessions.

For example, if the client believes that he/she cannot do any work in the midst of extreme anxiety or a panic attack, the experiment would be to try to do some work the next time severe anxiety is experienced. If a client feels that his/her spouse "would never understand my feelings" about anxiety (or some other issue), the client would be encouraged to try talking with the spouse about the issue.

Such behavioral experiments need to be individualized for each client. The outcome of the behavioral experiments will encourage the client to reevaluate his/her cognitions and beliefs. The focus of these behavioral experiments is to afford the client the opportunity to test the validity of beliefs and expectations about stressful situations. If the client places him/herself in the stressful situation to test out the predictions, then the client is also providing him/herself with an exposure trial.

At the beginning of each cognitive session, discuss the results of behavioral assignments from the previous week. Both you and the client should record the homework assignment on paper to increase the probability of compliance with the assignment. Remind the client to view stress and anxiety in daily life as providing opportunities to practice specific coping skills that have been learned. The client should try out all of the coping skills that have been presented and identify the strategies that are most helpful for him/her in different situations and for different stressors. Instruct the client to practice this assignment at least two times in the coming week. Instruct the client to record practices on the *Weekly Record* and mark those practices with an asterisk (*). Remind the client that the goal is to use both relaxation and cognitive strategies to deal with anxiety-arousing situations and thoughts. Remind the client to continue to monitor cognitions and to practice becoming more aware of cognitive errors.

C. Review and Planning

Briefly review errors in thinking, and reinforce the client's understanding of the cognitive treatment rationale.

Session 7

A. Session Goals

1. Review progress and problems on assigned practice items. Check practice session monitoring record and *Weekly Record* for accuracy.
2. Begin visualization practice with anxiety scenes (see Chapter 7).
3. Present self-instruction material.
4. Assign homework practice in a low-anxiety situation.

B. Session Procedures

1. Review the client's progress since the previous session. Be sure to check carefully for the success of the homework practices, and deal directly and expediently with any problems associated with the practices. Review the client's self-monitoring on the *Weekly Record* for accuracy and completeness. Be sure to recognize the client's efforts in keeping the records, and emphasize how important the record keeping and conscientious homework practice are for treatment progress.

2. Self-instruction. One method the client can use to overcome his/her fears and beliefs about entering an anxiety situation is training him/herself to use self-instruction. In this procedure, the client actively says to him/herself such things as, "You can continue working even if you are anxious." The use of self-instruction and autogenic phrases may at times help clients manage fears and anxiety about entering panic-associated situations or cue clients to look for alternative explanations in panicky situations. Suggest that the client develop a set of self-instructions that will likely be helpful and germane to the anxiety symptoms. If a client has difficulty developing self-statements, provide a list of examples (see Table 6-1) from which to choose two or three relevant statements. Instruct the client to write the relevant statements on 3″ × 5″ cards to which he/she can refer when noticing an increase in anxiety or fear that may signal a panic attack is approaching. Self-statements appear to be more effective if clients actually talk to themselves, either aloud or covertly, as opposed to simply reading the statements. In some instances, clients have found it helpful to audiorecord the statements and listen to the tape when necessary. Using role-play, modeling, and other in-office practice techniques may also be useful in helping the client learn how to use self-statements to manage panic-related problems.

A major focus of self-statements is to remind the client that he/she is in control of him/herself and that even in the midst of a panic attack, the client is in control of his/her behavior and body responses. Recognize that the client may be uncomfortable about deliberately placing him/herself in stressful circumstances; but by actively talking to him/herself, the client successfully can enter and stay in these situations. Point out that it is the confrontation with and realistic reappraisal of the stressful symptoms or situations that provide the most potent therapeutic effect. To the extent that the self-statements facilitate engaged exposure, they will be helpful adjuncts to treatment.

3. Assign a behavioral experiment in a low-level anxiety-provoking situation and ask the client to try using self-instruction to manage the

TABLE 6-1. Examples of Self-Statements

Coping Self-Statements
1. Stage of preparing for a stressor
   - What is it I have to do?
   - I can develop a plan to deal with it.
   - I can manage this situation.
   - No negative self-statements; just think rationally.
   - Don't worry. Worry won't help anything.
   - Remember that avoiding feared situations only makes my fears worse. I have to approach what I fear to learn to cope with anxiety.

2. Stage of confronting and handling a stressor
   - One step at a time. I can meet this challenge.
   - Don't think about fear, just about what I have to do. Stay relevant.
   - I can handle the situation.
   - This anxiety is what the doctor said I would feel. It's a reminder to use this situation as a way to learn to cope with anxiety.

3. Stage of coping with the feeling of being overwhelmed
   - Keep the focus on the present. What is it I have to do?
   - When fear comes, just pause.
   - I was supposed to expect my fear to rise.
   - I feel my fears rising and I accept that as a fact.
   - Let me label my fear from 0 to 10 and watch it change.
   - It's not the worst thing that could happen.
   - Don't run away.
   - If I stay here, in time my anxiety will certainly decrease.
   - This is an opportunity for me to learn to cope with my fears.
   - I can do what I have to do in spite of anxiety.
   - My anxiety won't hurt me.

Reinforcing Self-Statements
   - It worked; I was able to do it.
   - Wait until the group hears about this.
   - It wasn't as bad as I expected.
   - I made more out of the fear than it was worth.
   - My negative thoughts—that's a large part of the problem. When I control my negative thoughts and anticipations, I control my fear.
   - This experience will help me practice again in the future.
   - It's getting better each time I use the procedure.
   - I'm really pleased with the progress I'm making.
   - I can learn to overcome my fears!

Note. Adapted from Meichenbaum (1975).

situation. The client should be instructed to use both relaxation and cognitive coping strategies to deal with anxiety.

C. Review and Planning

1. Review the client's progress with relaxation and the cognitive coping strategies. Make sure the client fully understands that the purpose of using management techniques is to prepare for *in vivo* exposures and that while the managment techniques help them cope with anxiety, they may not eliminate the anxiety.
2. Review the *Weekly Record* and check that practice assignments were recorded on the bottom half of the the *Weekly Record*.

Session 8

A. Session Goals

1. Review the *Weekly Record* for accuracy.
2. Review progress in homework assignments.
3. Practice visualization with anxiety-provoking scenes.
4. Assign a homework assignment in a low-anxiety situation.
5. Present thought stopping and diversionary techniques for anxiety management.

B. Session Procedures

1. Check the *Weekly Record* for accuracy, and deal carefully, but expediently, with any problems associated with the homework assignment.
2. Spend approximately 20 minutes on visualization of anxiety hierarchy items (see Chapter 7). By now, the client should be visualizing items that produce moderate anxiety. Encourage the client to continue practicing visualizations at home and to practice both cognitive and relaxation techniques as often as possible throughout the next week.
3. With the client, develop the third behavioral experiment to be conducted *in vivo*. The assignment should focus again on a low-anxiety experience in order to help ensure that the client will be successful.
4. Thought stopping and refocusing techniques. Thought stopping and refocusing are designed to increase the client's control of both

thoughts and images. The basic idea is to cease dwelling on anxiety-provoking thoughts and images through self-control and/or refocusing one's attention. The client may be instructed to use anxiety-provoking thoughts and images as cues to stop ruminating, and to redirect his/her attention to relevant ongoing activities. For example, the client may be instructed to use an image, such as "a big red stop sign," to stop dwelling on the thoughts and images, and then to turn attention outward by becoming more fully engaged in the surrounding situation. In refocusing, instruct the client purposefully to direct attention away from catastrophic thoughts and images and toward the details of the tasks in which he/she is engaged. The client might focus on how well he/she is performing a task or how the client might improve task performance. Or at a business meeting the client might focus on how others in the situation are handling the stress.

Refocusing should help the client to become more fully engaged in the situation, not to pretend that he/she is not anxious or panicky. Rather, the purpose is to recognize the anxiety symptoms, but not ruminate about them. Therefore, caution the client that while refocusing may temporarily reduce anxiety in a specific situation, it should not be used as a way to avoid engaging in the experience. For example, the client should not pretend that he/she is not in the stressful situation. Nor should the client distract him/herself from bodily changes associated with anxiety or panic. Encourage the client to recognize the bodily change (e.g., increased heart rate) but not to linger on the catastrophic thoughts associated with the elevated heart rate.

C. Review and Planning

Review the homework assignment with the client. Make sure the client has blank *Weekly Record* forms. Remind the client to practice covert rehearsal as a way to increase skill with the cognitive coping strategies.

Session 9

A. Session Goals

1. Review the *Weekly Record.*
2. Review progress with homework assignments.
3. Continue visualization practice.
4. Assign homework assignments for moderate-anxiety situations.

B. Session Procedures

1. Review the *Weekly Record* with the client, and discuss the results of homework assignment.

2. Spend approximately 30 minutes practicing visualizations of moderate-anxiety items with the client.

3. Develop the next homework assignment. This assignment should be for a moderately anxiety-provoking situation. However, use your own clinical judgment as to whether the client should either repeat a low-stress assignment or move to a moderately stressful assignment.

C. Review and Planning

Review the homework assignments with the client, and remind the client to practice relaxation and visualizations at home in the coming week. Check for any problems that the client is having with the treatment protocol.

Session 10

A. Session Goals

1. Review the *Weekly Record.*
2. Review the homework assignment.
3. Continue visualization practice.
4. Assign homework assignment in a moderately anxiety-arousing situation.

B. Session Procedures

1. Review the *Weekly Record.* Discuss what the client has learned through the use of the record, and emphasize the importance of the record as a learning device. Discuss the results of the homework assignment and explicitly check on the client's use and facility with the cognitive coping skills.

2. Spend approximately 30 minutes practicing the visualization procedures with items from the anxiety hierarchy (see Chapter 7). Be sure to discuss the client's use of cognitive coping strategies and cue-controlled relaxation during these exercises.

3. Develop the next homework assignment. This assignment should be in a moderately anxiety-provoking situation for the client; however, use your own clinical judgment as to whether the client is ready to complete *moderate anxiety* homework tasks. This decision should be based on an assessment of the success or failure of previous homework assignments and the client's readiness to move to more stressful situations.

C. Review and Planning

Make sure the client has sufficient blank *Weekly Record* sheets. Remind the client to practice visualizations at home. Review this week's homework assignment. Give the client the opportunity to verbalize any problems with treatment.

Session 11

A. Session Goals

1. Review the *Weekly Record* and the client's progress.
2. Review the homework assignment.
3. Practice cue-controlled and cognitive coping strategies with imagery.
4. Assign the next homework assignment.

B. Session Procedures

1. Review the *Weekly Record* and the client's progress in the previous week. Check that the client is practicing visualizations and anxiety-managment skills. Discuss the effects of and problems with these techniques. Discuss the results of last week's homework assignment. Keep in mind whether the client is ready to move on to more difficult assignments.
2. Spend approximately 30 minutes practicing covert rehearsal with the client. If you deem it appropriate, have the client practice high-anxiety hierarchy items. Work carefully to uncover negative thoughts and images; elaborate cognitive coping strategies.
3. Allow the client to design this week's homework assignment. This assignment should be a *high*-stress situation for the client; however, use

your own clinical judgment as to whether the client is ready to cope with a high-anxiety situation. Base this decision on an assessment of the client's previous success or failure during previous homework assignments, as well as the client's readiness to move to more anxiety-inducing situations.

C. Review and Planning

Make sure the client has blank *Weekly Record* sheets for the coming week. Remind the client to practice visualizations at home. Review the homework assignment with the client.

Session 12

A. Session Goals

1. Review the *Weekly Record* and the client's treatment progress.
2. Review the homework assignment.
3. Practice cognitive coping strategies.
4. Assign a homework assignment in a high-anxiety situation.

B. Session Procedures

1. Review the *Weekly Record* and the client's progress in the previous week. Discuss the results of the preceding homework assignment at length, particularly if a high-anxiety assignment was attempted. Encourage the client to view the assignment as a success experience even if the results were not what the client had envisioned.

2. Spend approximately 30 minutes practicing coping imagery with the client. By now, the client should be practicing high anxiety items. Because this is the last session in which imagery will be practiced, try to complete the hierarchy. Encourage the client to continue practicing the imagery at home. If the client has not practiced all hierarchy items by this session, urge him or her to try to complete the remaining items at home.

3. Allow the client to design a high-anxiety homework assignment. However, again keep in mind that you must use your own clinical judgment as to whether the client is ready to attempt such an assignment. Spend some time helping the client prepare coping strategies to complete the assignment successfully.

C. Review and Planning

Remind the client to continue practicing imagery at home. Review the homework assignment. Make sure that the client is not experiencing any problems with treatment that have not yet been brought to light. Remind the client to continue to practice and use the relaxation skills.

Session 13

A. Session Goals

1. Review the *Weekly Record* and treatment progress.
2. Review the homework assignment.
3. Begin generalization practice.

B. Session Procedures

1. Review the *Weekly Record*. Make sure the client is continuing to record on them accurately. Note the situations that have been problematic for the client, as you may use this information later in this session. Review progress and problems.
2. Review the previous week's homework assignment. Encourage the client to tell you what was learned from the experience.
3. Generalization practice. The following two treatment sessions are designed to help the client generalize coping strategies to a greater variety of life situations and to integrate the cognitive coping strategies with the *in vivo* exposure treatments. In a sense, the homework assignments have served as initial *in vivo* exposures. At this point in treatment, you make such work explicit. Begin the session by working with the client to summarize the range of situations in which the client has made progress in coping with and controlling anxiety. Then say something like the following:

We see that you have made progress in dealing with anxiety in a variety of situations in your life. By applying the strategies we discussed here in the office, you have made changes where it counts—in your life. I hope you understand the importance of practicing what you have learned here in real-life situations. It is only by facing the situations—and your anxiety—that you gain control over them. Learning what situations or cues initiate "false alarms" for you and how to deal with those "false alarms" has been a central focus of therapy. In our remaining sessions, we are going to work together to devise ways for you to continue your progress in therapy on your own. One way to begin to do that is to begin to apply your coping skills to more situations in your life. We will do this by conducting behavioral experiments specifically designed for that purpose.

Each situation in your life in which you find yourself experiencing anxiety is a new opportunity for you to practice exposing yourself to stressful situations and coping with the interfering thoughts and symptoms. Confronting situations that you have already mastered is very important also. Each time you practice in new situations you extend the range of control you have over your panic symptoms, and you decrease the probability that a "false alarm" will occur.

Use examples from the client's treatment progress to show how *in vivo* practice has helped the client gain mastery in controlling panic attacks. Point out how risks taken in real-life situations have benefitted the client.

I can't emphasize enough the importance of practicing your skills in all the situations that produce anxiety for you. Practice is crucial in keeping and increasing the gains you are making. Many research projects show that practice is a powerful factor in improvement. Practicing skills in new situations is helpful in another way: It helps reduce anxiety about panic—that "fear of the fear." Each time you can enter a situation and tolerate your anxiety, you fear your panic in the situation less. Remember that what you have learned here is a set of skills. Like all skills, they improve with practice. Dedication to practicing your skills in different situations will help you gain mastery over anxiety in more of your life.

Then, work with the client to design a generalization practice. If you think the client is ready, this should take the form of a high-anxiety homework assignment specifically designed to tackle a relatively new practice situation. For example, a client who is afraid of panicking when dealing with authority figures may elect to have lunch with his/her boss, if this is something the client has not done. Then guide the client to understand that such an assignment gives the client the opportunity to widen the range of life situations with which he/she can cope. Be careful to help the client select an assignment that probably can be managed successfully. The first generalization practice should not be too dissimilar to tasks successfully completed in the past.

C. Review and Planning

Encourage the client to verbalize his/her understanding of the importance of practice in various situations. Remind the client that it is also important to continue coping with anxiety in the situations already improving with practice. All practice is good—in both old and new situations. Review the homework assignment. Make sure the client has blank *Weekly Record* sheets.

Session 14

A. Session Goals

1. Review the *Weekly Record* and treatment progress.
2. Review the homework assignment.
3. Continue generalization practice.
4. Begin planning future practices.

B. Session Procedures

1. Review the *Weekly Record* and the client's progress in the previous week.

2. Review carefully the results of the previous homework assignment. Encourage the client to recognize the value of the assignment in terms of generalization. If there were problems with the assignment, help the client identify aspects that still were mastery experiences. If the client was very anxious, point out that it is only by experiencing anxiety that we learn to control it. Explore the negative hypotheses the assignment disconfirmed.

3. Work with the client to schedule several more generalization practice homework assignments for coming weeks, which the client will complete through his/her own efforts.

C. Review and Planning

Review this week's homework assignment and make sure the client has a written copy of the schudule of future assignments. Remind the client that the next session is the last one. Be sure to assure the client that the clinic will maintain contact with him/her after treatment ends in order to follow up on the client's continued treatment progress.

Session 15: Generalization Practice and Termination Issues

A. Session Goals

1. Review the client's progress in treatment.
2. Remind the client to continue practicing on a daily basis.
3. Review treatment progress and give instructions for the next 6 months.
4. Schedule the posttreatment assessments.

B. Session Procedures

1. Inquire as to client's general status as well as success with homework assignments. Review the practice monitoring sheets.
2. Review the *Weekly Record* for accuracy as well as for signs of specific problems that have developed for the client.
3. Briefly review the cognitive procedures and rationales used during this treatment program, focusing most on those procedures that have been most useful to the client. Include comments on the following:
   a. The three-response model of anxiety and the role of "false alarms" in panic symptoms
   b. The importance of using coping procedures to facilitate continuing exposure to fearsome situations
   c. Automatic thinking
   d. Analysis of faulty logic
   e. Decatastrophizing
   f. Exploring alternatives
   g. Reattribution
   h. Rescue factors
   i. Hypothesis testing
   j. Self-statements
4. Because this is the client's last therapy session, generally review the client's progress in treatment and attend to termination issues. Instruct the client to continue to use the coping strategies he/she has learned during treatment, and encourage the client to continue to assign homework activities for him/herself. Remind the client that the clinic will contact the client for 6- and 12-month follow-ups, but if the client has questions about therapy progress or procedures or runs into a situation with which it is difficult to cope, he/she should feel free to telephone the clinic. Also, mention that if necessary, the clinic is, of course, available

for crisis intervention. Schedule the client for posttreatment assessment, and remind the client about formal 6- and 12-month follow-ups.

C. Review and Planning

Spend some time dealing with any unresolved termination issues and solidifying rapport with the client. Encourage the client again to practice the coping strategies on a daily basis and in as many different situations as possible in order to maximize generalization. Remind the client again about follow-up assessments.

Check to make sure that all of the necessary data have been collected and that the client's needs to have been met as well as possible within the framework of this protocol. Remind the client that continued practice is necessary to maintain gains and continue improvements.

7

Exposure Treatment Component

Exposure therapies are both refinements and elaborations of a behavior therapy technique originally termed *flooding*. "Flooding treatments," in turn, are essentially clinical applications of experimental procedures developed in laboratory paradigms of neurosis and avoidance learning. Kazdin (1978) traced the roots of flooding procedures beginning with Masserman's (1943) work with induced neurotic reactions to cats. Masserman showed that by forcing cats to remain in a situation in which they had previously received shock, the cat's attempts to escape from the fearful situation would eventually diminish. Subsequently, laboratory research with animals confirmed that persistent avoidance responses could be extinguished if the fearful stimulus was presented continuously after the avoidance response was made. Likewise, preventing an animal from escaping from a fear stimulus would also extinguish the fear responses conditioned to that stimulus situation. While various conceptual models have been suggested as operative mechanisms to explain why prolonged exposure to fearful stimuli functionally eliminates anxiety reactions to those stimuli (see Barlow, 1988), none of these models seems to be adequate as an explanation of the success of the exposure procedures. On the other hand, what seems to be perfectly clear from a large body of research is that prolonged exposure to a fearful situation does facilitate the elimination of fearful and panic-like responses to those fearful situations.

Exposure therapy refers to procedures in which a patient exposes him/herself to a fear-evoking stimulus, either in real life (*in vivo* exposure), in fantasy (imaginal exposure), or in some structured but artificial situation (*in vitro* exposure—for example, a clinical laboratory or a therapist's office). Clinical research has suggested that exposure treatments should be (1) prolonged (rather than of short duration),

(2) repeated until all the anxiety and fear associated with the situation is eliminated, (3) graduated from low-stress to high-stress situations, and, of course, (4) clearly specified—that is, planned (Emmelkamp, 1982; Mathews et al., 1981).

In addition deSilva and Rachman (1981) have argued that not just any form of exposure to fear-inducing stimuli will lead to fear reduction. Rather these authors maintain that the client has to be engaged in the exposure situation. Engaged, or active as opposed to passive, exposure requires that the client attend to and interact with the feared stimulus rather than directing attention away from the feared stimulus.

And finally, Borkovec and Sides (1979) have suggested that exposure treatments will be more successful if the exposure trials actually provoke symptoms of anxiety. The latter suggestion is certainly in keeping with deSilva and Rachman's recommendation that the client be actively engaged in the fearful situation as well as with Lang's (1977) suggestion that including response propositions as well as stimulus propositions in imagery exposure will lead to the optimum effect.

While the preceding suggested guidelines for doing exposure treatments have been generally accepted among clinicians, and, in fact, provide the guiding structure for the exposure treatments included in this therapy manual, more recent research has questioned the necessity or at least the essential nature of these guidelines. For example, deSilva and Rachman (1981) have suggested that while prolonged exposure to fearful situations may be a sufficient condition for fear reduction, there is no good reason to suppose that such exposure is a *necessary* condition for fear reduction.

More recently, Rachman, Craske, Tallman, and Solyom (1986) tested the hypothesis that escape behavior strengthens agoraphobic avoidance responses. In this study, patients were either instructed to remain in the fearful situation until there was a substantial reduction in their anxiety (the standard approach in prolonged exposure trials) or to leave the exposure situation while their anxiety was at a peak level. The results of the study showed that escape responses were followed neither by increases in fear nor by decreases in estimates of control or safety in the situation. Consequently, the authors concluded that escape from anxiety-provoking situations does not necessarily strengthen agoraphobic avoidance responses.

While these studies seem to call into question the necessity of some of the procedural components suggested for exposure treatments, they do not suggest necessarily that these components should be eliminated from the exposure procedures. In addition, as both Butler (1986) and Rachman (1983) have noted, the aforementioned exposure procedures basically are guidelines rather than scientific principles because the underlying mechanisms of exposure therapies are not at all well understood. On the other hand, these procedures have been shown to be very effective in the treatment of various anxiety disorders.

Application of exposure therapy to panic disorder requires some modification of the standard procedures. In the case of agoraphobics and simple phobics, there generally are fairly clear-cut environmental situations (i.e., external situations), around which planned prolonged exposures can be arranged. While it may be that some cases of panic disorder also present with clear environmental avoidance responses, in the vast majority of the cases, panickers experience their panic attacks as "coming out of the blue" and not especially associated with any particular external environmental situation. Consequently, arranging exposure situations for panic-disordered clients requires some additional modification of the usual procedures.

Whereas in many phobic situations, we conceptualize the treatment as exposure to an external stimulus, in the case of panic disorder we think of the exposure in terms of exposure both to external *and* to internal fear-associated stimuli. That is, the cues that provoke the panic responses in panic-disordered clients are not necessarily based in the external environment but rather are, in at least some cases, internal somatic or physiological stimuli that cue the fear response (see Chapter 2). While these internal somatic cues may be functionally related to either behavioral or external environmental conditions, their relationship to these behavioral or external conditions is not easily manifested. In addition, the internal somatic cues may be of such short duration and/or low frequency that arranging prolonged exposure becomes difficult at best. In this regard, both panic disorder and social phobias share a common element. In work with social phobias, Butler (1986) suggested several exposure strategies that may be relevant to the treatment of panic disorder, such as the development of a graduated hierarchy of panic-associated situations.

Developing a graduated hierarchy of panic-associated situations may be difficult initially because panic clients typically have not associated their fear with specific stressful situations; nor have they considered that their somatic responses themselves are the relevant cues. Usually careful self-monitoring of panic attacks will suggest at least some items for the hierarchy. If common themes pervade panic situations, then hierarchies can be constructed around those themes. For example, if hectic work schedules, dramatic temperature changes, or physical exertion are associated with panic, then hierarchy items can be constructed around these themes, all of which may be functional in a wide range of specific situations.

Another possible solution is to construct the hierarchy according to the frequency or durations with which an item is practiced. For example, rapid breathing may produce panic symptoms and if practiced at high frequency or for a long duration, they may be very anxiety-arousing. If practiced at low frequencies or for short durations, the activity would fall much lower in the hierarchy. Thus, the number of repetitions or the length of the exposure might provide a basis for hierarchy construction.

Remaining actively engaged in the exposure situation appears to be a critical element in exposure treatments. Active engagement may be facilitated in several ways. First, clients should write out in as much detail as possible the exact plan for the exposure trial *and* carry the assignment with him/herself during the practice for easy reference. The plan should specify behaviors (e.g., maintain eye contact, listen carefully, count your breathing rate) that will help direct the client's attention to the relevant practice cues. Whatever the planned exposure behaviors are, they have to be structured in such a way as to maximize the probability that the client will complete the assignment. Besides using the graduated hierarchy, we also encourage clients to use their newly learned relaxation skills and cognitive coping strategies as aids toward completing the assignments. However, we caution our clients not to use the management skills to distract their focus away from the exposure tasks.

Finally, provoking symptoms of anxiety not only helps assure that active engagement is taking place but also helps ensure that the patient is exposed to the relevant internal (somatic) stimuli that often cue the fear response in panic patients. To this end, we have instituted the *in vitro* exposure component of our therapy package. To the extent that clients identify and practice behaviors that provoke some somatic cues in the office, they will be in a better position to attain full value of the *in vivo* exposures. In fact, it may be that active engagement in an exposure trial is defined by the presence of all three behavioral components—namely, behavioral, cognitive, and physiological responses.

Within our integrated treatment package, exposure treatment begins in the sixth therapy session. By this time, clients should be well on their way to mastering relaxation skills and proficient enough with the cognitive strategies to be aware of the attentional factors as well as any cognitive avoidance responses that might attenuate the effects of the exposure procedures. Of course, practicing relaxation itself often begins the internal exposure process because of the sudden physiological changes and resulting loss-of-control sensations in panic patients during initial relaxation exercises, as noted in Chapter 5. Again, the exposure component is but one of the three major treatment elements in the total package. While presented separately here, in our clinic, exposure procedures are added to and integrated with the other components.

Session 6

A. Session Goals

1. Present the rationale for exposure therapy.
2. Develop exposure hierarchy.

Therapist Reminder. This session begins the full application of all three panic treatment components. Up to Session 6, clients have been learning relaxation skills and cognitive coping strategies as panic and anxiety management procedures. Now the goal is to begin to use those anxiety-management skills in planned exposure trials. Planned exposure will take place in three forms: imaginal exposure, *in vitro* exposure, and *in vivo* exposure. It is important to remind the client that while the management techniques are helpful in reducing anxiety levels, by themselves they probably are not sufficient to reduce panic attacks. Management skills are helpful in panic treatment to the extent that those skills increase the probability that clients will complete the planned exposure therapies.

B. Session Procedures

1. Rationale for exposure therapy

As you may recall from our earlier meetings, we feel that panic attacks are essentially "false alarms" issued by the body in response to a cue or signal that you have learned to associate with danger or threat. The problem, of course, is that these panic alarms are, in fact, false. Nevertheless, the fear associated with the panic attacks is quite real. Just as false alarms are learned phenomena, the treatment for them also involves planned relearning experiences. The term we use to describe these corrective learning experiences is *exposure therapy*.

The basic logic of exposure therapy is quite simple. Exposing yourself to those situations and cues that have been associated with anxiety and panic attacks provides you with the opportunity to learn at least three things: (1) You will learn that anxiety and panic symptoms can be controlled using the relaxation and cognitive coping techniques that you have been learning. In fact, you will learn that you are able not only to reduce those troublesome symptoms, but also actually to bring them on at will. (2) You will learn that there is no basis for the fear associated with your panic attacks. (3) And, finally, you will learn to break the association between the cues that signal your fears and panic attacks and teach yourself new ways of responding during graduated exposure to those panic-associated cues.

At the present time, we do not fully understand the exact mechanisms that explain how this new learning takes place, but we do know that exposure therapy is highly effective in treating anxiety disorders. Let me emphasize that it is the new learning that takes place during exposure trials that is the critical element in therapy. The exposure to panic-associated cues merely provides the opportunity for that learning to occur. Therefore, passive exposure to these same cues—that is, unplanned exposures during which no corrective learning takes place—is not sufficient to bring about therapeutic changes in your behavior. During the exposure trials we encourage you to deal directly with your anxiety and fear and to take an active part in the new learning process.

Because you will be exposing yourself to these anxiety-provoking cues, you should anticipate that initially you may become more anxious and perhaps notice an increase in panic attacks. However, as you know, in most cases, anxiety and panic attacks are self-limiting—that is, in most situations the anxiety and/or panic symptoms will subside. The anxiety and fear itself, of course, may be quite unpleasant.

In order to minimize the amount of unpleasantness you will have to experience, we will develop together a graduated hierarchy of anxiety-provoking cues and work through that hierarchy from the least to the most anxiety-provoking situations. Nevertheless, it will be necessary for you to tolerate some anxiety, at least initially, as you learn to deal more effectively with anxiety and panic symptoms and to eliminate "false alarms," you should notice substantial reductions in the number and perhaps intensity of your panic attacks.

There are three ways that you can expose yourself to panic-provoking cues. First, you can imagine yourself experiencing the panic-provoking situation or cues. Imaginal exposure provides not only an exposure trial under controlled and low-arousal conditions, but it also allows you rather easily to plan and practice your management skills in imagination so that you will be prepared to take full advantage of *in vivo* exposures. Second, you can expose yourself to certain panic-provoking cues here in the office. We will explore ways to induce those bodily sensations that have come to signal the possibility of a false alarm. And, finally, you will be exposing yourself to actual situations in your daily life. Today, we will begin with imagery training and hierarchy development.

2. During this session, train the client in imagery visualizations by instructing the client to visualize neutral and/or pleasant scenes. Explain that during future sessions, he/she will be visualizing personally relevant stressful scenes, but that first it is important to practice how to visualize.

Introduce imagery training in a fashion similar to the following:

I am now going to task you to imagine some scenes. The kind of imaging I am going to ask you to do is like daydreaming, except that you will control it more. As you know, some daydreams can be quite vivid. Sometimes you may feel like you are really there. Try to imagine these scenes that vividly. Picture the scene in your mind as clearly as you can.

The first scene will involve drinking a glass of water. As I present the scene to you, try to visualize the scene with as much detail as you can include, just as if it were real. Try to involve yourself fully in the scene as an active participant. Imagine yourself moving as you would move if you were really drinking. Feel how thirsty you are before you drink, and how good the water tastes. Notice how clear and cool the water is. Do everything you can to make the scene real. Now I will present the first scene. As I describe it, create the scene in your mind. When I finish the description, keep imagining the scene until I tell you to stop. Here is the first scene. (*Be sure to read slowly.*)

You walk into a square, blue room. The walls and ceiling are all a deep blue. On the floor is a blue carpet. The carpet is soft under your feet. There is nothing in the room except for a plain wooden table in the middle. On the table are a clear glass pitcher filled with water and a tall, clear glass. You are thirsty, and you are glad to see the water. Your mouth is dry. You walk over to the table and pick up the pitcher in one hand and the glass in the other. You fill the glass with water. Your hand holding the glass feels cool as the glass fills with water. You set the pitcher back down on the table and move the glass to your lips. The water cools your whole mouth and refreshes your whole body as you take the first swallow. You drink the whole glass of water.

Wait 60 seconds or so, and ask the client about the experience. Ask if the client actually saw the scene and felt the sensations described. If the client did, respond with praise; if the client did not, explain that imagery skills can improve with practice. Obtain a clarity rating (on a scale of 0 to 8; see scale later in this chapter), and repeat vividness instructions if necessary. Say something like the following to the client:

I'd like now to practice with another scene. This involves sitting by the window in the sun. Again, try to picture all the objects in the scene as thoroughly as you can, and try to feel with your body what you really would feel. Here is the scene. You are sitting by a window. The window is square, with one unbroken pane of glass. There are yellow and white checkered curtains on the sides. You are sitting on a soft chair; you feel comfortable and relaxed. Your elbows are on the window sill, and your hands are clasped under your chin. The sun is streaming through the window onto your face and arms. You feel warm, and the light is bright. You close your eyes and feel the warm sun.

Again, wait 60 seconds or so and discuss the experience with the client. Ask if the client actually saw the window and felt warmth, felt the soft chair, etc. Obtain a clarity rating, and repeat vividness instructions if necessary. Say something like the following to the client:

Let's try one more scene. In this one, you will be walking uphill on a warm day. Try to see the hill and everything in the scene; try to feel what is happening to your body. It is late spring. You are walking up a hill. You are on a dirt path lined with tulips and lilacs. The tulips are bright purple and the lilacs are white. You can smell them in the wind. The day is hot, and your feet feel tired. The ground is soft and not easy to walk on. You begin to sweat a little bit, and you rub your forehead with the back of your hand. The back of your hand feels wet. You get close to the top of the hill, and you begin to hurry. You can feel your heart pound as you get to the top. At the top is a soft patch of grass, in the shade of a tree. You sit down on the grass and rest. You look at the path with the purple tulips.

Discuss the experience. Ask if the client saw and felt the scene, with particular attention to heart sensations. Following each scene, ask the client to rate how clearly the scene was visualized on a scale of 0 to 8 as follows:

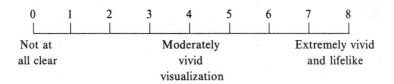

If the clarity rating is still below 4, repeat one of the scenes with the client. Give the client a sheet on which the three scenes are written. Tell the client to practice imagining the three scenes once a day for the next week. In addition, tell him/her that, as an additional exercise, each evening the client is to imagine a scene of something that happened that day. Tell the client to pick a pleasant or neutral scene. Remind the client to try both to see and to *feel* the sensations experienced during the scene—that is, where possible, to try to recreate the sensations and responses of the actual experience.

3. Hierarchy development. Following visualization practice during this session, develop an individualized 10-item anxiety hierarchy with the client. Because most clients do not avoid situations, hierarchy items should be rated on a scale of 0 to 8 in terms of the degree of panic

typically elicited by or associated with the situation. Include in the hierarchy situations that range from low levels of anxiety (ratings of 1–3) to high levels (ratings of 6–8), as well as situations that exemplify different types of stressors relevant to the client. One such hierarchy is presented in Chapter 8. Inform the client that the situations included in the hierarchy are examples of situations that the client encounters that provoke or are associated with anxiety and that these items will be used in future sessions to learn how to cope with stress and anxiety and to reduce panic episodes.

Hierarchy items should include both external environmental (situational) stimuli (e.g., hectic work situations, being alone, being criticized or observed, receiving an injection) *and at least one* hierarchy item focusing on one or more salient anxiety symptoms—that is, an internal stimulus (e.g., tachycardia, dizziness, palpitations, breathing difficulty). Ideally, the internal symptoms should be associated with elicitation or provocation of anxiety or panic attacks.

Note that the purpose of the imaginal exposure sessions is to help prepare the client for *in vivo* exposure. Because fearful or distracting thoughts may keep the client from fully attending to and/or engaging in the exposure situation, it becomes imperative that the client learn to change these negative thoughts to facilitative plans of action. Our experience suggests that it is not necessary to teach the client that such thoughts have to be eliminated but rather to practice how to deal with such thoughts because these negative thoughts may interfere with their receiving full benefit from the *in vivo* exposure. All hierarchy items, whether internal or external, need to be described in sufficient specific detail so that clear and vivid visualization is possible.

C. Review and Planning

1. Review the visualization procedures with the client, and instruct the client to practice visualizing a neutral or pleasant scene *at least* three times during the next week. Each practice should focus on just one or two scenes, and the client should continue the practice until he/she is able to visualize the scene vividly—that is, at least a 4 or 5 on the scale of 0 to 8.

2. The client should reflect on the content of the anxiety hierarchy during the next week, noting any modifications he/she feels may be appropriate for the hierarchy. These changes should be discussed during the next session.

Session 7

A. Session Goals

1. Attempt panic symptom induction.
2. Train in diaphragmatic breathing.
3. Complete the first trial of imaginal exposure.
4. Assign self-directed exposure in a low-level anxiety-provoking situation.

B. Session Procedures

1. Review the client's success with the visualization practices conducted at home. Ensure that the client is able to visualize neutral and pleasant scenes clearly and vividly. In some cases, additional in-office practice may be necessary before the remaining therapy procedures can be started.

2. Review the anxiety hierarchy, incorporating any changes the client may have thought of since the previous session. Be sure that the client is satisfied with the hierarchy while recognizing that the hierarchy is likely to change over the course of time.

3. Introduction and rationale of breathing exercises: Hyperventilation example.

a. First, provide a general overview of breathing problems, along with the following rationale.

Incorrect breathing practices are often found in people with anxiety problems. Even if you are not one of those persons who has problems breathing correctly, changes in breathing patterns that could account for some of the anxiety that you experience are a normal response to fear or high anxiety. Therefore, we can safely assume that, at least when you are experiencing high anxiety, you experience changes in regular breathing patterns. It is important, therefore, that you learn proper breathing techniques as part of your set of skills to deal with anxiety.

Most people associate huffing and puffing kinds of breathing patterns with hyperventilation. However, there are other breathing patterns that can result in hyperventilation. These include such things as shallow breathing and other irregularities, such as sighing a great deal or holding one's breath and then trying to compensate by taking in large volumes of air.

The most common irregularities are important for you to recognize because the symptoms of hyperventilation, including difficulty breathing, tingling sensations, pain in the chest, numbness, and others, are very similar to those experienced with panic attacks. These physical sensations then become cues that a panic-prone person interprets as the beginning of a panic attack; that is, these sensations cue the onset of fear that an anxiety attack is starting, and the fear in turn elicits a physical response—namely, release of epinephrine (adrenaline) and other hormones that, of course, intensify the physical symptoms.

This sequence of physical reactions elicited by fear is a perfectly natural body response, and it is adaptable when one finds oneself in a dangerous situation. In regard to anxiety attacks, however, there is no apparent dangerous situation. Rather, becoming aware of a change in your physical status (e.g., dizziness or tachycardia) serves to cue a fear response—namely, "I am having an anxiety attack," which starts the whole process into action. The initial change in physical status may be due to things like exercise, excitement, temperature changes, hyperventilation, and so on, but they serve as cues to elicit a "whole body" anxiety attack.

What I'd like to do now is give you an example of what can happen with hyperventilation. Hyperventilation is not the only way to elicit these feelings, nor does it work for every person, but now I want you to test out how hyperventilation affects you. I want you to try breathing rapidly and shallowly through your mouth for a few minutes. When you begin to feel the symptoms I've described or others that you associate with anxiety, I want you to describe them to me.

Have the client breathe rapidly (25–30 breaths/minute) for a maximum of 3 minutes. As soon as the client signals that he/she experiences symptoms, record these symptoms and instruct the client in methods to correct any breathing problems. At this point, it may be useful to ask clients to identify any other somatic cues or behaviors that consistently signal anxiety or an impending panic attack. The objective here is to identify as many (internal cognitive, physiological, and behavioral) cues that induce or are associated with panic attacks. These cues should, wherever possible, be integrated into the exposure hierarchy.

It is not atypical for these cues to be highly idiosyncratic and/or unrecognized by the client. For example, one of our clients, who was a high school teacher, complained of frequent panic attacks during his third-hour class. He reported the panics always started for no apparent reason and usually only at the beginning of this class. He insisted there was nothing different about this class; in fact, this was perhaps one of his best classes.

After several unsuccessful attempts to identify possible cues for his panic attacks, the therapist requested that the client tape-record the activities of this class during his next panic attack. As the therapist reviewed the audiotape, the client provided a narrative of his actions. Shortly after calling the class to order, there was a long silence during which the client indicated he was becoming tense, anxious, and "feeling like the panic was going to hit any second." This silent period was followed by the teacher's instructions to the class to complete an assignment from the textbook. The client explained that because of his panic attacks he had learned to prepare such assignments so that he could avoid having to try to lecture during panic attacks. The therapist asked what the client was doing during that long initial silence. He responded that he had been taking attendance, which was the responsibility of third-hour teachers. The therapist asked the client to demonstrate how he took attendance. During this demonstration, the client reported the same sensations that he experienced at school, namely anxiety and dizziness. The client came to recognize that the up and down head movements he made as he glanced from the class to his attendance cards was associated with the dizzy feelings. By using the same rapid head movements, he was able to reproduce in the office the panic-precipitating sensations. We then incorporated this internal cue of dizziness into the exposure hierarchy.

b. Instruction in breathing techniques. Two specific techniques are implemented in order to slow down breathing and to develop diaphragmatic breathing methods. Instruct the client to place one hand on the upper chest and one on the abdomen, with the little finger of his/her hand just above the navel. Clients are to attempt to "balloon" out the stomach while attempting to have as little movement as possible of the hand placed on the upper chest. Demonstrate this procedure to the client, and attempt to aid the client in successfully following this procedure. If the client is unable to do this procedure perfectly, encourage successive approximations, and inform the client that "this procedure will take practice, but with practice in ballooning out your stomach to attain diaphragm breathing, you will also be able to slow down your breathing." Then instruct the client to attempt to stretch out a breathing cycle to a count of about 8 seconds. This can be 4 or 5 seconds breathing in and 3 or 4 breathing out. "Think of the process as if you were pouring thick oil from one drum to another. This will help you make the breathing cycle as smooth and fluid a motion as possible."

Have the client attempt to do both techniques as one exercise. For those clients who are unable to slow breathing, tell the client either to try a 5- or 6-second cycle and work toward 8 seconds or to try silently saying, "*Pause, relax*," in between each breathing cycle. If the client is still unable to approximate diaphragm breathing, instruct the client to lie on the floor, face down with both hands under the head. This position makes thorax breathing very difficult and for many clients may be a necessary first step.

Try lying on the floor, on your stomach, with your arms crossed and supporting your head. This will help you learn to breath correctly or at times when it is especially difficult for you to control your breathing. While first learning these techniques, it may also be helpful to lie on your back and place a light book or piece of paper on your stomach, then attempt to move the book or paper up and down as you breath. The book or paper simply helps you to monitor your abdominal movement.

Attempt to practice the slow, diaphragmatic breathing technique during that part of the relaxation exercises when the word "relax" is paired with deep breathing. Combining diaphragmatic breathing with relaxation is another step toward eliminating the habitual onset of anxiety that is cued by the sensations associated with irregular breathing practices. In addition, you should begin to use the diaphragmatic breathing and relaxation exercises when you experience mild anxiety. As you become more skillful in these techniques, you will find them very helpful in controlling your anxiety. Although you are just beginning to learn the skills you need, it would be helpful to start attempting to use them to reduce low levels of anxiety.

Continue, in following sessions, to reinforce applying these techniques whenever the client experiences anxiety and as another coping technique.

4. *In vitro* exposure to internal panic-associated cues affords the client the opportunity to learn (a) that at least some of the internal physiological sensations can be induced behaviorally and/or cognitively and (b) that these responses can be modified or controlled by adaptive behavioral changes. While these in-office exposures may be therapeutic themselves, the full impact of exposure therapy is best accomplished *in vivo*. To the extent that *in vitro* exposures move the client along toward full *in vivo* exposure, the technique is helpful.

In our clinic we have found that imaginal exposure to anxiety-provoking thoughts and panic behaviors; voluntary rapid breathing; physical activities such as running in place, spinning in a chair, chest constriction; noticeable temperature changes; exposure to bright light (e.g., overhead florescent lights); and occasionally catastrophic thoughts may elicit the frightening physical symptoms associated with panic attacks. Our opinion is that any number of changes in behavior or physiology, manifest or not, may elicit panic symptoms. Which cues elicit panic-like symptoms may be less important than demonstrating to the client that such feelings can be elicited in a very subtle fashion that often escapes awareness and that these feelings can be changed. After assessing which induction procedures most reliably elicit at least mild levels of panic symptoms, these procedures should be included in the imaginal exposure hierarchy as well as practiced in the office.

The purpose of the *in vitro* exposure is to help desensitize clients to the fear associated with these panic-associated cues. Emphasize to the clients that panic attacks that seem to occur spontaneously may actually be cued by these internal, somatic responses, which are induced by changes in the client's external or internal environment. Because the client is not aware of or focused on those environmental changes, the sudden increase in anxiety seems to "come out of the blue." The in-office use of behaviors that may induce the panic-associated cues seems to be a powerful therapeutic tool that demonstrates well how previously unexplained spontaneous panic attacks might, in fact, be quite explainable and brought on or terminated at will. Clients seem to learn quickly how to identify such environmental changes and how to adapt to such changes once the interoceptive model is conceptualized clearly.

Either rapid breathing or chest constriction can bring on panic-like symptoms; but, as noted, a fairly large number of behaviors or stimulus situations, some of which may be highly idiosyncratic, are also useful in this regard. The therapeutic problem is to identify and isolate those cues. If attempts at inducing panic-like symptoms using the preceding situations fail, hints of more idiosyncratic experiences may be gleaned from the *Weekly Record* sheets.

Initially, have the client engage in the panic-symptom-inducing behavior for several minutes in the office. Ask the clients to rate how closely the induced sensations match those experienced during a panic attack, and instruct the client to become more aware of how such sensations might be induced in other situations. These *in vitro* demonstrations also provide a convenient format for discussing feelings of loss of control and how such perceptions of loss of control might exacerbate the panicky feeling. How often *in vitro* practices are done in therapy sessions varies tremendously from client to client. Try to incorporate the specific cues into the imaginal hierarchy, and have the client practice these cue-inducing behaviors, where possible, during both imaginal and *in vivo* exposure.

5. Begin the anxiety visualization practice using the following procedures:

a. Have the client recline in a chair and use relaxation skills to get as comfortable as possible. Instruct the client to visualize scenes as vividly as possible (as if he/she were really in the situation) and to maintain visualizations until instructed to stop. To make scene descriptions more powerful, place emphasis on the client's response propositions (i.e., on vivid descriptions of the client's responses), especially somatic and emotional responses associated with anxiety. To this end, try to incorporate the *in vitro* induction procedures into the imaginal exposure hierarchy. If such integration is not possible or not effective, then separate *in vitro* practices may be necessary. If the client experiences anxiety (level of 2 or greater) during visualization, he/she should (1) raise a forefinger and keep it raised until the anxiety decreases below 2; (2) rehearse coping with the anxiety through the application of cognitive coping strategies and relaxation skills. After considering the client's skills level and readiness to employ the skills in anxiety-arousing situations, use your judgment to determine whether coping skills (and which ones) should be used in this session.

b. If the client does not signal anxiety, each visualization should be 60 seconds long.

c. If the client does signal anxiety, instruct the client to continue visualizing the scene and to attempt to cope with the anxiety through the application of coping strategies. Periodically remind the client to focus on anxiety, maintain the visualization, and practice applying coping skills.

d. When the client lowers his/her forefinger to indicate that anxiety has ended, continue the visualization for another 60 seconds, then terminate the visualization.

e. The maximum length of each visualization should be 10 minutes, even if anxiety has not decreased by this time. (*Exception*: If client finds it impossible to maintain an image for this amount of time or if the hierarchy item involves a very brief, discrete situation—e.g., experiencing a heart palpitation—the maximum length of visualization can be reduced to 5 minutes.)

f. After each visualization, inquire and record information about the following: clarity of image, maximum level of anxiety, coping strategies used (getting details about the way in which cognitions were changed, the situation was reevaluated, etc.), and anxiety level subsequent to use of coping strategies. A form for recording this type of information (Therapist Record: Imaginal Exposure Practice) can be found in Appendix D. Discuss with the client any problems encountered and ways of improving the ability to cope with anxiety. Record the relevant information.

g. The criterion for moving up to the next hierarchy item is two consecutive 60-second visualizations in which anxiety is not signaled at all. (If criterion has not been reached after five visualizations, return to preceding hierarchy item or revise hierarchy item so that it is less difficult.)

h. Special problems during visualization:

• In some instances, the client may report no increase in anxiety during visualization because of a failure to reproduce the negative thoughts usually associated with that situation, rather than successful use of coping strategies; such a situation becomes apparent during the inquiry. If this happens, prompt the client by saying, "The next time you imagine this scene, include both the negative thought you usually have in that situation and the coping strategies you would use."

• If the client *begins* the session with an anxiety level of 2 or above (some clients report resting levels of 2 or above), then the client should be instructed to signal if anxiety *rises* above resting level during visualization (1 full point or more) and lower finger when anxiety returns to resting level. Note both the resting level and the amount of change on the record form.

6. Review the client's success with the previous session's homework assignment. (See Chapter 6, Session 6. Recall that the first homework assignment was given as a "behavioral experiment" to test the client's ability to cope with interfering cognitions. We now use this one brief practice to build the first self-directed *in vivo* exposure.) Present self-directed *in vivo* exposure trials in a graduated fashion, beginning with low-stress situations. As well as possible, try to choose assignments that have a high probability of success; however, perhaps more important is choosing assignments that are meaningful for the client.

Together with the client, *write out* a specific homework assignment that can be practiced *at least* twice before the next session. Ideas for exposure trials may come from the client's imaginal exposure hierarchy or from situations that the client expects to occur during the next week. Situations likely to occur only one time during the forthcoming week will not suffice because at least two practices are necessary, and preferably more. Tell the client that the more he/she practices, the more proficient he/she will become at mastering the anxiety management techniques and the more new learning will occur during the exposures.

Encourage the client to remain in the stress situation as long as possible and until he/she notices a substantial reduction in anxiety (at least a 2-point reduction on the anxiety rating scale of 0 to 8 or until the panic attack subsides. If, in the situation, the client does not find him/herself becoming anxious, encourage him/her to use rapid breathing, chest constriction, or whatever behavior has been used in the clinic to bring on the feelings or somatic sensations associated with panic attacks. If the client experiences anticipatory anxiety sufficient to motivate avoidance behavior, then he/she should use both relaxation and cognitive coping strategies to reduce the anxiety or panic symptoms to the point at which the exposure trial can be initiated. These same management techniques can be practiced during the exposure trial to reduce premature escape from the exposure situation. During the exposure trial, caution the client not to focus attention away from the panicky feelings or from the demands of the ongoing exposure activities. Try to help the client to become and remain fully involved in the exposure activity.

One example of such a low-anxiety-arousing exposure trial is provided by a client who was an ardent golfer. This woman complained of one to four "spontaneous" panic attacks per week. Rapid breathing in the office reliably produced the lightheadedness she experienced during panic attacks. Her exposure hierarchy included a wide range of stress-related situations in which she had experienced panic attacks, including driving in traffic, a tightly scheduled work day, walking alone in a park, being in crowded hot places, relaxing at home, and playing golf.

She worked in an executive sales position, one which required entertaining clients. A round of golf usually allowed her to combine business with pleasure. She was quite a good golfer, who found the game relaxing; however, she had several panic attacks while playing golf, after which she found herself becoming tense, anxious, and less productive during golf outings, although her pleasure in the game remained high. She reported having her first golf-related panic attack during a company golf outing. The panic occurred on the tee of a short hole that forced play to slow down and forced the foursome behind hers to wait and watch as she and her foursome teed off. She had already been tense because she was playing in a foursome with two business associates she had just met. As the time for her tee shot approached, she had a panic attack, which forced her to explain that she was not feeling well, to apologize to her playing partners and to leave the course.

After this incident, she found that she was tense and anxious while golfing and had difficulty concentrating on either her golf game or her business clients, primarily because of her fear that she might again panic on the course. She reported several "little panics" in similar circumstances, but none of these limited symptom attacks prompted her to escape from the golf course. She gave a rating of 2 to the item "playing golf with business associates."

Her first self-directed exposure assignment was to schedule at least two business rounds of golf during the following week. During the golf game she was to focus—as usual—on her golf game, and if necessary use her coping skills to control her anxiety level. If she panicked during the match, she again was to use her coping skills and continue to play on. In any case, she was *not* to engage in behavior that distracted her from either her anxiety or her golf game (i.e., she was not to pretend that she was not anxious, nor was she to disengage herself from conversations with her playing partners). Rather she was to redouble her efforts toward her play and her interest in her partners discussions. In addition, she was to note whatever new learning took place for her, including which coping strategies worked best for her in that situation. The client wrote the assignment on a 3" × 5" card that included notes to herself. She carried the card with her during the trial. The result of each exposure trial was transferred to her *Weekly Record* as a practice trial. From this practice the client learned that continued engagement in the ongoing activities facilitated reductions in her anxiety and increased her confidence that the treatment would be helpful.

C. Review and Planning

1. Remind the client that the purpose of the coping skills is not to "fight the anxiety" but rather to keep the anxiety at a manageable level, allowing the full extent of exposure therapy to take place. Thus, the client should not try to prevent anxiety from developing; in fact, he/she should welcome anxiety as an opportunity both to practice management skills and to receive the full impact of exposure therapy. Only in this way will the client learn to break the association between the onset of anxiety cues and the fear of panic attacks.

2. Make sure that the client fully understands the homework assignments and has a written copy of the assignment.

3. Remind the client to continue completing the *Weekly Record* and practice records for the management skills.

Sessions 8–15

A. Session Goals

1. Continue the imaginal exposure and *in vitro* procedures.
2. Continue self-directed *in vivo* exposures.

B. Session Procedures

During each of Sessions 8–12, conduct both imaginal and *in vitro* exposure according to the protocol described in Sessions 6 and 7. For imaginal exposure, the goal is to work through the graduated hierarchy from lowest-to highest-rated scenes. For most clients, four sessions should be sufficient to complete the hierarchy, although a few (usually the more severe cases) may take six or more sessions to complete the hierarchy. A key issue here is staying focused on the task. Combining the exposure treatment with cognitive and relaxation therapy does not leave much time for you to explore interesting problems or personality dynamics that may become manifest during treatment. Clearly, crisis situations as well as problems that may interfere with consistent progress in therapy have to be dispatched efficiently. This is especially the case for Sessions 6–9, during which the protocol structure will take almost the full hour to complete.

It takes a good deal of clinical expertise to decide which are crisis situations that need immediate attention and which are problems that can be dealt with at a later time. Try to deal with nonprotocol problems that develop during therapy by incorporating the problem into the treatment protocol. For example, family problems may present an opportunity to apply relaxation or cognitive skills to a new situation, or perhaps a homework assignment can be designed to help deal with the problem. It is not unusual that non-panic-related problems crop up in treatment and need to be handled. On the other hand, this panic treatment protocol is not sufficient to deal with all such possible problems. Occasionally it may be necessary to refer a client for some other type of additional therapy (e.g., family therapy). Provided that the different therapies are coordinated, we find such arrangements quite satisfactory.

Continue exposure to internal panic cues in the office until the client exhausts his/her list of potential internal panic-eliciting cues. As the client discovers each such cue, he/she practices it during the session, and wherever possible incorporates it into the graduated imaginal hierarchy. In addition, encourage the client to use these internal cues (e.g., rapid breathing, muscle constriction, cognitions) to exacerbate or induce anxiety during self-directed *in vivo* exposure. Essentially, this suggests to the client that he/she actively attempt to increase anxiety during self-directed exposures. Point out to the client that one way to solidify treatment gains is to overlearn the treatment procedure. To the extent that self-induced anxiety provides additional opportunities to overlearn coping skills and cues that help discriminate reality-based alarms from false alarms, such experiences are helpful. Because the therapeutic intent is to have the client become anxious during the practice trials, anxiety-cue induction is *not* used as a paradoxical intention, in which the hope is that the client will *not* become anxious when he/she tries to.

Self-directed *in vivo* exposure homework is assigned on a weekly basis beginning with Session 7. Low-level anxiety-provoking situations are assigned for homework for the first two self-directed exposure trials. The third and fourth self-directed exposure trials are built around moderately (3–5 rating) anxiety-arousing situations. And, finally, highly anxiety-arousing situations are prescribed for exposure. For most clients, this sequence works well. The objective, of course, is to move to the most distressing situations as quickly as possible without overwhelming the client with unmanageable anxiety or panic attacks. Use both the data provided by the client about success with previous exposure assignments and good clinical judgment to gauge the difficulty of exposure assignments.

While it is preferable that the client complete the exposure homework on his/her own accord, for some of the more difficult cases it may be helpful for the client to ask another person to accompany him/her during the exposure trial. If this type of aid is helpful, it should be limited to the first exposure practice trial and at least two additional practice trials should be completed unaccompanied. Reliance on others to complete the exposure trials should be discouraged as soon as possible. Continued insistence on such accompaniment may suggest that the assignments are not appropriate, the schedule is moving too quickly, or perhaps, that the protocol is not appropriate for the client.

The last two scheduled treatment sessions (14 and 15) are used to deal with termination issues and to plan continued in vivo exposure practices. With the client, develop additional and, where possible, novel experiences to which the client can continue to expose him/herself after treatment ends. Insist that the client write these generalization experiences in a chronological list, such that at least two generalization exposure trials are scheduled each week for the 8 weeks following termination. Thereafter, encourage the client to continue practice on his/her own accord and to record each practice in a diary. Tell the client again that he/she may encounter stressful situations that elicit panicky feelings. Encourage the client to see such occasional panic episodes as good opportunities to practice the panic management skills in unplanned exposure trials. Remind clients that you will be contacting him/her to arrange 3-, 6-, and 12-month follow-up interviews, at which time you expect to share the practice entries from the client's diaries. Also encourage the client to contact the clinic should the client experience a significant increase in panic episodes after treatment ends. But also tell the client that research shows that most clients, in fact, not only maintain gains made during treatment but, in most cases, continue to improve, especially for those who continue to practice and use the skills learned during treatment.

8

Case Illustration

The case illustration in this chapter should help both to clarify how we integrate the three major components of our panic treatment package and to provide more concrete examples of the procedures discussed in previous chapters. The case history, that we have chosen for this chapter was selected because it represents a clear and relatively straightforward application of our panic treatment program. We do, however, hasten to add that this is not necessarily a typical case of panic disorder nor is it the most difficult case in which the panic treatment program has been used at our clinic.

Unlike most of our cases, this client presented with a relatively acute onset of panic attacks. In the vast majority of the cases that present at our clinic, clients report a long and chronic history of anxiety problems. On the other hand, as with many of our clients, this individual had been treated by several physicians for various kinds of possible medical problems, including anxiety. He was referred to our clinic by a cardiologist to whom he had presented with concerns about cardiac functioning.

Also, like the vast majority of our clinic clients, this client had multiple diagnoses. However, his additional diagnoses were given severity ratings of 3 (on our severity scale of 0 to 8), which is below the minimal clinical severity level of 4 (i.e., a severity level below 4 is a problem judged not severe enough to need treatment at the present time). Thus, while this client's primary diagnosis was panic disorder, the diagnosticians also noted that there appeared to be features of other DSM-III diagnoses.

Finally, as with a large percentage of clients referred to our anxiety disorders clinic, this client was using medication (alprazolam, 2.5 mg, three times a day) at the time of the diagnostic interviews. He agreed to withdraw from the medication under medical supervision before treatment was initiated. Many of our more chronic cases are far more reluctant to withdraw from medication before treatment begins. We generally prefer our patients to be off of psychotropic drugs before treatment so that we are better able to assess clearly the type and extent of the client's problems and the client's response to our treatment. However, psychopharmacological withdrawal is *not* a prerequisite of our treatment program. When clients using medication begin our treatment program, we coordinate our efforts with the client's physician. In the majority of cases, clients reduce the medication use or stop using medications entirely by the time treatment ends.

Background

Mr. P was a 39-year-old white, married, male with two sons, aged 13 and 4 years. This was the first marriage for both Mr. P and his wife, who worked as a part-time secretary. Mr. P completed 2 years of vocational training as a machine tool-and-die specialist after completing high school. For the previous 20 years, he had been employed with the same large industrial firm. During the ADIS interviews, Mr. P complained that he felt anxious, tense, and nervous approximately 75% of his waking hours. The tension and anxiety had begun approximately 3 months before the first diagnostic interview. In addition, his general anxiety and tension was punctuated by three or four full-blown panic attacks per week. The majority of the panic attacks occurred either as he was just entering sleep or upon waking from sleep. During the panic attacks, his major symptoms included tightness in the chest, general muscular tension, tachycardia, paresthesias, and general agitation.

Fear of dying and/or losing control during his panic attacks were prominent cognitive features. For instance, during a panic attack he insisted that he was going to have a heart attack and constantly wondered how long the panic attack was going to last. He reported that he has had panic attacks while sitting in a chair trying to relax, while reading the newspaper relaxing, while trying to nap or sleep, while shopping, and at work. Although he felt that the panic attacks were related to cumulative stress in his life (e.g., dissatisfaction with his job and general stress associated with raising his children, especially his 4-year-old child), he was not aware of any particular cues that elicited the panic attacks. On the other hand, he was aware that when he felt more stress (i.e., when he was having a "bad day"), it seemed as though he were more likely to have a panic attack.

His first panic attack occurred approximately 3 months earlier while he and his wife were out shopping. He reported that the shopping trip had been quite pleasant as they looked to buy some new furniture for their home. As they were shopping in a furniture store he suddenly felt nauseous, weak, and dizzy, and he experienced chest tightness, chest pressure, and dyspnea. He described the situation as one in which he felt like he was about ready to pass out. Being a volunteer fireman, he attempted to take his pulse which he could not find and suddenly thought he must be having a heart attack, and, in fact, that his heart had "stopped." His wife and the salesman helped him lie down on the floor and an ambulance was called. He was taken to the emergency room of a local hospital, where the physician on duty diagnosed esophagitis that triggered a fainting spell.

Mr. P did not agree with the diagnosis and insisted that during the panic attack his heart had ceased to function for at least a brief period. He was discharged from the hospital emergency room, and the following week made an appointment with his own physician for a medical exam. The results of the medical exam were negative. For the next several weeks he had almost daily panic attacks and almost constant anticipatory anxiety associated with the fear of having another panic attack. Because of the severity and the frequency of his panic attacks, he returned to his physician, who prescribed alprazolam for him. While the medication seemed to decrease somewhat the intensity and the frequency of his panic attacks, the panic attacks continued at the rate of about three to four a week. Consequently, Mr. P went to see a cardiologist, who found no physical basis for his complaints and referred him to the Anxiety Disorders Clinic.

Mr. P did not recall any particular life stress at the time that his first panic attack occurred. Although he did recall that about a week before his first panic attack he had to go to the roof of his home to make some repairs and while he was on the roof he became very tense and anxious because he had a mild fear of heights. This client, who was really quite insightful, also recognized that he could exacerbate his anxiety symptoms by focusing his thoughts on the fear of dying and/or losing control during the panic situation.

Mr. P's medical history was essentially negative, with the exception of chronic lower back pain that was associated with his work situation. He had been troubled with back pain for approximately the preceding 10 years. He reported that his father had been alcoholic, although his father had never been diagnosed or treated for alcoholism. He also said that his mother had both a pronounced fear of heights and "nervous problems" that as far as he knew were neither diagnosed nor treated. He reported that his father's brother also had "nervous problems" and had attempted suicide for which he had been hospitalized. Except for the preceding, there were no other reported instances of psychiatric problems in the family. In the week between the two diagnostic interviews, Mr. P completed a battery of questionnaires and a *Weekly Record* so that by the time of the second diagnostic interview, 2 weeks of the *Weekly Record* were available to the diagnostician. The results of the questionnaire data and the *Weekly Record*, as well as the Hamilton Anxiety and Depression scores, are presented in Table 8-1 and Figure 8-1. After the second diagnostic interview, Mr. P received the following DSM-III consensus diagnoses: panic disorder, severity level 5 (on a scale of 0 to 8); simple

TABLE 8-1. Mr. P's Scores on the Pretreatment, Posttreatment, and Follow-Up Assessments

Measure	Pretreatment	Posttreatment	6-month follow-up
BECK	13	4	6
CSAQ-C	20	15	15
CSAQ-S	24	11	15
DYAD	104	105	101
EYS-E	15	8	16
EYS-N	14	14	10
EYS-L	3	3	5
FQT	15	11	11
FQS	5	1	1
PSSS	71	41	50
STAI-S	57	36	24
STAI-T	48	42	49
HAM ANX	28	8	11
HAM DEP	22	7	11
Clinicians' ratings	5	2	0

Note. BECK = Beck Depression Inventory; CSAQ-C = Cognitive Somatic Anxiety Questionnaire—cognitive score; CSAQ-S = Cognitive Somatic Anxiety Questionnaire—somatic score; DYAD = Dyadic Adjustment Scale; EYS-E = Eysenck Extraversion score; EYS-N = Eysenck Neuroticism score; EYS-L = Eysenck Lie score; FQT = Fear Questionnaire total fears; FQS = Self-rating from the Fear Questionnaire; PSSS = Psychosomatic Symptom Scales; STAI-S = State–Trait Anxiety Inventory—State score; STAI-T = State–Trait Anxiety Inventory—Trait score; HAM ANX = Hamilton Anxiety score; HAM DEP = Hamilton Depression score; Clinicians' ratings = average ratings from two independent clinical raters, based on a clinical interview.

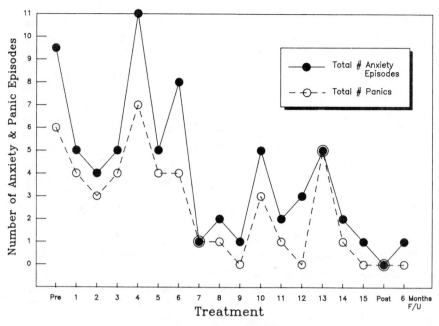

FIGURE 8-1. Case study data.

phobia of heights, severity level 3; generalized anxiety disorder (GAD), severity level 3.

Treatment

Session 1

During the first therapy session, the client was presented with the standard rationale for the treatment program, and the treatment schedule was explained to the client. In addition, the therapist reviewed the client's history and presenting complaints. The therapist also reviewed with the client the results of the self-monitoring from the *Weekly Record* sheets. The client's second week of pretreatment recording is displayed in Appendix A.

During the review of the *Weekly Record*, the client stated that much of his stress apparently was associated with his job, his job schedule, and the management of his 4-year-old son. He also recognized that he had "perfectionistic tendencies," which increased the stress in his life. The therapist noted that the patient appeared to be quite optimistic about the treatment approach, especially about the use of relaxation and cognitive techniques to manage the panic and anxiety in his life.

Sessions 2 and 3

The second therapy session began with a review of the client's *Weekly Record* from the previous week. The data on the *Weekly Record* indicated that Mr. P had had five panic attacks during the previous week, all of them occurring around sleep time or during sleep. The duration of the panic attacks averaged 5 minutes, with a range from 1 to 15 minutes. The client also had reported that he had one limited symptom attack that occurred in one of his classes related to being a volunteer fireman.

After a quick review of the *Weekly Record* for the previous week, the therapist introduced the 16-muscle-group relaxation training session. The therapist then went on to provide the foundation rationale for the cognitive coping skills, during which the therapist called attention to the "comments column" of the *Weekly Record* and suggested that the client might start noting any cognitions that occurred during or immediately preceding panic or anxiety episodes. In response to that suggestion, the client quickly noted that during panic attacks he focused his attention on the possible physical consequences of having an anxiety attack, namely, that he feared he would drop dead or lose control of his behavior, which would make him "look bad" to others. The therapist reemphasized the importance of monitoring not only his physical symptoms but also the cognitions that he was having during panic attacks.

By the third therapy session, Mr. P was reporting that while the frequency of his panic attacks seemed to be stabilizing, the intensity of the panic symptoms, especially the somatic symptoms, seemed to be attenuating somewhat. The majority of this client's panic attacks seem to be occurring at times he was either falling asleep or awakening from sleep. During this session, the 16-muscle-group relaxation with discrimination training was presented per the protocol. The therapist noted that the client seemed to be able to understand as well as put into practice the fundamental relaxation procedures with some facility. In addition, the client reported that he had found that the relaxation practices helped facilitate his falling asleep at night.

Following relaxation training, the therapist continued to present didactic material on exploring alternatives and reviewed cognitive monitoring procedures. The client was able to demonstrate his comprehension of the didactic material by relating his fear of having a panic attack while around his colleagues either at work or at the volunteer fire station. These thoughts were especially stressful for him because he felt that it would be obvious to everyone around him that he was anxious and consequently he would be embarrassed.

Sessions 4 and 5

During the fourth and fifth therapy sessions, Mr. P continued to report doing well but had data reflecting a marked increase in anxiety (see Figure 8-1). The majority of both of these sessions was spent focusing on cognitive didactic material. The analysis of faulty logic was introduced and explored in sufficient detail to allow the therapist to assess the client's comprehension of the material. In addition, the presentation of didactic material on decatastrophizing, rescue factors, reattribution and hypothesis testing were all presented per the protocol outline. The therapist relied heavily on material recorded in the client's *Weekly Record* to demonstrate, elaborate, and make concrete the concepts that were presented didactically. In Session 4, the 8-muscle-group relaxation with discrimination training was practiced, and it was repeated in Session 5. By this time, the therapist had noted that the client seemed to have developed quite well the ability to employ the relaxation skills both at home and during breaks at his job.

Daily relaxation practice forms (see Appendix C) reflected this fact. As can be seen, anxiety ratings were dropping consistently during relaxation, and relaxation ratings reflected somewhat increased relaxation as a result of the practice. Nevertheless, comments recorded during practice sessions reveal that some anxiety and discomfort was occurring on occasion during these sessions.

Data from Figure 8-1 indicate quite clearly that Mr. P was experiencing his highest levels of anxiety and panic. In fact, Mr. P also reported increasing his medication usage in order to deal with increased anxiety. More careful inquiry revealed a situation that we see quite often. By focusing on anxiety and panic, he found himself thinking more about the experience of anxiety and the somatic symptoms associated with it. Relaxation exercises also served to focus attention on his somatic symptoms. Thus, Mr. P seemed to experience an episode of relaxation-induced anxiety somewhat later than is usually the case with clients proceeding through this protocol. As noted in Chapter 5, these experiences are seldom dramatic when relaxation procedures are taught under the direction of a therapist. The most severe examples of relaxation-induced anxiety or panic occur when patients attempt these exercises alone.

Nevertheless, it was important to observe increased anxiety at this point in time and relate it to his focus of attention on somatic interoceptive cues.

Session 6

By the time the sixth therapy session was scheduled, the client seemed to be well on his way toward mastering the relaxation skills as well as demonstrating a fundamental grasp of the cognitive monitoring procedures and the basic rationale for the entire treatment program. At the sixth therapy session, 4-muscle-group relaxation training was introduced and practice in imagery skills was accomplished. In addition, the initial exposure hierarchy was developed. Mr. P's exposure hierarchy is presented in Table 8-2. In Tables 8-3a and 8-3b, we present additional examples of exposure hierarchies to emphasize the broad range and idiosyncratic nature of these hierarchies. Initially, Mr. P was able to elaborate only seven items for the exposure hierarchy. In later sessions, however, he was able to detail several more hierarchy items, and he was able to refine and elaborate on some of the original hierarchy items.

On several of the items in the hierarchy, we incorporated somatic responses that were prominent during this patient's anxiety attacks— namely, tightness in the chest, difficulty breathing, palpitations, and feelings of dizziness. Wherever possible, we tried to emphasize the response propositions involved in the situations as well as the external stimulus cues in the situation.

The review of the client's *Weekly Record* at the sixth therapy session indicated that the frequency of his panic attacks had decreased by about 50% over preassessment. However, some anxiety episodes were still high, due (seemingly) to stress at work. The therapist reviewed some of the didactic material on errors in thinking and again reminded the client of the importance of continuing his good efforts in self-monitoring anxiety and panic attacks.

Session 7

The protocol schedule for the seventh therapy session is quite busy; consequently, this session has to be executed expediently. Review of the client's *Weekly Record* showed that he had only one panic attack during the previous week, and the attack lasted for approximately 15 minutes. Unlike the majority of his previous panic attacks which, occurred around

TABLE 8-2. Mr. P's Imaginal Exposure Hierarchy

Item	Anxiety rating (0–8)
1. Working in the garden, hurrying to complete a task before nightfall. Fatigue from a long work day makes your muscles feel weak and tired.	2
2. The older son teases the 4-year-old son, and a screaming match develops between them. The noise from the screaming makes the vessels in my head throb and I can feel myself becoming tense.	3
3. Working the best I can on my job, but my boss doesn't recognize how hard I am working and proceeds to make unreasonable demands on me. I can feel the muscles in my arms, chest, shoulders, and neck tense up.	4
4. Arguing with the assistant chief at the firehouse during a practice drill. My leg and arm muscles feel weak because of the required physical exertion. I can hardly talk, and it is difficult to breathe.	5
5. Feeling frustrated because of my back and shoulder pain that keeps me from doing what I want to do. I feel stiff and weak and think that I am becoming an invalid.	5
6. During the day, there is a fire alarm, and I have to stop whatever I am doing and hurry off to the fire. At the sound of the alarm, I can feel my heart speed up, and the tightness and pressure in my chest makes my muscles ache. I begin to sweat and have difficulty breathing. I have to force myself to move.	6
7. I am trying to relax and watch a ball game on the TV. I've just put my 4-year-old to bed, but he won't stay in bed and keeps on crying and calling to me. He won't give me a minute's rest. I can feel the tension building in my neck and head. I am losing my patience with him, and the anxiety level is building. I wonder if it's going to get so bad that I'll have a panic attack.	6
8. I am working at home and suddenly my heart starts to pound and the heart rate increases. I feel a pressure and tightness in my chest, and I can feel the panicky feelings starting to rush on. I know something is wrong with me but I don't know what it is.	7
9. As I wake up in the morning I am aware of tightness in my chest; my heart is pounding, and I have difficulty breathing. My muscles ache they are so tense. I feel sweaty and afraid to move. I feel so weak I probably could not move if I wanted to. I can feel the vessels in my head and legs throb with each heart beat.	8
10. Trying to fall asleep with difficulty. There is a general uneasiness; I can't relax. I can feel my chest tightening up, and I start to breathe faster and faster. My heart starts to pound and I feel weak and lightheaded. I get very warm and start to sweat heavily. I wonder if my heart is going to stop.	8

TABLE 8-3a. Example of an Exposure Hierarchy Developed by a 39-Year-Old Attorney with a 1-Year History of Panic Attacks in a Wide Range of Situations (Diagnosis: Panic Disorder)

Item	Rating (0–8)
1. Feeling incompetent to speak up in a meeting with colleagues	3
2. Feeling lightheaded and dizzy while eating dinner in a hot, noisy, restaurant	4
3. Theatre—afraid of panicking and feeling like I have to leave; stomach cramps and fear that I will lose control of bowels	4
4. Waking up in middle of night and stay in same bed—afraid that I will panic (pounding heart, difficulty breathing) if I don't move to another room; no concern with gastrointestinal problems in my own home	4
5. Hyperventilating—experiencing difficulty breathing, dizziness, and palpitations	4
6. Attending business meeting—afraid I won't be able to concentrate, will want to leave; afraid I will run out of room or won't be able to get to bathroom in time	5
7. Asking a request of an employee—afraid of their refusal; that is, assertiveness and afraid of losing the friendship	6
8. Attending night classes—feeling trapped, afraid of losing control of bowels, but sticking it out	7
9. Stay in motel room with family—feel trapped, afraid of feeling trapped, heart palpitations, diarrhea	8
10. Remembering panic attack in courtroom—difficult to leave; felt heart racing, sweating, gastrointestinal problems, and strong urge to run out	8

TABLE 8-3b. Example of an Exposure Hierarchy for a 41-Year-Old Woman with a 2-Year History of Panic Attacks and Concerns about Pregnancy (Diagnosis: Panic Disorder)

Item	Rating (0–8)
1. Coming to therapy sessions to talk about anxiety problems	2
2. Meeting an old friend unexpectedly and feeling uncomfortable talking about myself	3
3. Having to talk with my husband's ex-wife about anything	4
4. Having to do a daily ovulation test	5
5. Waiting for the results of a pregnancy test	6
6. Feeling lightheaded and as if I am going to faint while in church	7
7. Going to a reproductive endocrinologist for an examination	7
8. Finding out I am pregnant	8
9. Experiencing prolonged palpitations	8

sleep time, this attack occurred unexpectedly during the day. The client reported that when the panic attack started, he immediately instituted his relaxation and cognitive coping strategies to help manage the panic. He felt quite successful in being able to deal with the panic symptomatology. These reports helped document that the client was putting to good use the management skills that he learned in the treatment sessions and suggested that the client was ready to begin the exposure component of the panic treatment protocol.

During the seventh therapy session, 4-muscle-group relaxation training was repeated. A good deal of time was spent discussing the rationale and the utility of hypothesis testing and the use of cognitive coping strategies in difficult situations. The majority of the seventh therapy session, however, was spent in practicing the imagery visualization procedures and exploring panic-symptom-induction techniques. The therapist presented the material on diaphragmatic breathing training, to which the client responded most enthusiastically. The client noted that during the relaxation training, the use of controlled breathing to deepen relaxation levels was particularly helpful to him, and he appreciated the additional material on breathing training. The imagery visualization training was completed, with the client claiming good clarity ratings. Time did not permit initiation of the imaginal exposure treatment.

For homework, the client was asked to practice the breathing training techniques along with cognitive coping strategies at least twice in order to facilitate sleep induction. The client was specifically instructed to keep track of either self-statements or other cognitive strategies, for example, reattribution statements or recognition of rescue factors that would facilitate sleep induction. A particular focus of this homework assignment was to test the hypothesis that the client would be able to fall asleep despite a stressful and/or hectic day.

Session 8

The eighth therapy session began with imaginal exposure and an explanation for the rationale for self-exposure homework assignments. The first anxiety hierarchy item was completed, with the client reporting a rise of only one point in anxiety during the visualization. At this point, the therapist halted progression of imaginal exposure and introduced panic induction in order to demonstrate not only that panic symptoms could be induced by behavioral methods but also to provide the patient with another method of producing panic-associated somatic symptoms during exposure. It is our feeling that this response enhancement during exposure increases the effectiveness of exposure treatments. Therefore, the therapist explored with the client in greater detail the kinds of somatic responses that the client felt during panic or heightened-anxiety situations.

Referral to the previous *Weekly Record* provided good examples that helped the client recall some of the symptomatology during panic attacks. The most consistent symptom appeared to be his experience of chest tightness. Because attention had been focused on breathing techniques, he also reported that he tended to use shallow breathing rather than diaphragmatic breathing during periods of stress or anxiety. Therefore, the therapist began by having Mr. P breathe rapidly (at about a rate of 30 breaths/minute) and shallowly in the office. After approximately 40 seconds of rapid breathing, the client reported that he was beginning to feel somewhat lightheaded, anxious, and diaphoretic. The therapist instructed the client simply to return to diaphragmatic breathing and to try to relax for a few seconds. When the client was again in a stable state, the therapist explored with the client the extent to which the symptoms he felt with rapid breathing matched those he felt during states of panic. While clearly the intensity of the symptoms experienced with the anxiety-elicitation procedure was lower than that in panic situations, the client did report that they were somewhat similar to the symptoms experienced during a panic attack.

He noted, however, that in addition to the symptoms experienced with rapid breathing, he also routinely experienced a tightness in his chest that was not present with the rapid breathing. Therefore the therapist then had the client practice chest expansion (taking a deep breath and holding it). This technique proved to be fruitless in eliciting anxiety symptoms. The therapist then suggested that the client attempt chest constriction by simply letting all the air out of his lungs and then wrapping his arms around his chest and pulling as tightly as he could to exert pressure on his chest. The immediate response of the client to this procedure was one of immense surprise in terms of how similarly this chest compression technique matched his feelings of tightness and heaviness in his chest during a panic attack.

The therapist then combined rapid shallow breathing with chest constriction in an attempt to demonstrate to the client how the somatic symptoms he experienced during panic attacks could be brought on by these two procedures. The combination of these two techniques was highly successful in bringing on a rather strong anxiety reaction which the client said was quite similar to, although less intense than, the kinds of experiences he has during a panic attack. At this point the therapist had the client practice these *in vitro* panic-evocation procedures again and suggested that the client use the responses generated by these procedures to elaborate on his imagery during imaginal exposure. Although not yet revealed to the client, the therapist realized that these procedures may also be helpful in *in vivo* exposure trials in order to help elicit anxiety responses.

The therapist returned to the first imaginal exposure hierarchy item and again had the client imagine that item with elaboration of somatic responses. If necessary, the client was asked to incorporate shallow breathing into the hierarchy item. When this was done, the client reported a substantial increase in anxiety (3 points on our scale) to the first hierarchy item. Once the client had indicated the increase in anxiety, the therapist suggested that the client employ relaxation and cognitive coping strategies to help reduce the anxiety.

After repeating the first imaginal exposure hierarchy item, the therapist turned attention to discussion of hypothesis testing and the utilization of cognitive coping strategies during stressful and panic-like situations. The client was encouraged not only to monitor more carefully the cognitions during stressful and panic situations but also to pay particular attention to the breathing pattern during panic situations. The therapist asked the client to try to note any additional somatic symptomatology that occurred during the panic attack or that might signal a panic attack.

Finally 4-muscle-group relaxation training by recall was practiced. The review of the client's *Weekly Record* took place at the end of this therapy session and was used primarily not only to check on the client's progress but also to point out instances that had occurred during the previous week in which the client could have practiced both relaxation and cognitive coping strategies. Together, the client and the therapist decided that evocation of anxiety by means of chest tightness and shallow breathing was to be practiced at least twice during the next week. In addition, during times of stress and/or panic or anxiety attacks, the client was to continue to practice cue-controlled relaxation and to try to use as many of the cognitive coping strategies as he found helpful.

The symptom-evocation homework assignments were to be conducted with a second goal of testing the hypothesis that an activity could be completed in spite of anxiety or stress in the situation. That is, while the client was involved in some activity (e.g., gardening), he was to elicit the panic symptomatology and at the same time try to continue on with his activity. *After* he had come to some decision about whether or not he could continue on with his activity in the face of the anxiety symptomatology, he was to practice his management skills in order to reduce his tension and anxiety.

Session 9

During the ninth treatment session, the therapist began by reviewing the previous week's homework assignment and *Weekly Record*. Mr. P reported no panic attacks during the previous week and only one episode of moderate anxiety-evocation practices. He reported that he continued to use his cognitive coping and relaxation skills with great success not only to decrease anxiety but also to help reduce his general stress levels. While the client reported that he was rather successful with the use of cognitive strategies, the therapist noted that the client was not particularly facile in recognizing "errors in thinking" or being particularly aware of automatic thoughts associated with increased stress and anxiety. Consequently, the therapist took this opportunity to review the didactic materials on thinking errors presented during earlier sessions and again encouraged the client to read the handouts at home at least several times during the next week.

The role of diversionary cognitive strategies to avoid or control anxiety during homework assignments was then discussed. The therapist emphasized that during *in vivo* exposure trials, the client was not to engage in cognitive activities that would take his attention away from the total experience or that would allow him to avoid completely experiencing the anxiety reactions during the exposure trials. The rationale for self-directed *in vivo* exposure was again emphasized to the client and the use of the anxiety-provocation procedures to amplify the exposure trials was also reviewed. In addition, the therapist and the client together explored other kinds of behaviors that might be associated with panic cues. For example, the client noted that extended physical exertion, especially if he were fatigued before the activity began, would also usually lead to elevations in his anxiety levels, and in stressful situations, to panic attacks. Consequently the therapist suggested that times of physical exertion might be an appropriate opportunity to practice anxiety management skills and may also provide an ideal arena for exposure practices.

The next two items on the imaginal exposure hierarchy were then completed in this therapy session. Each of these items required four presentations before the criterion was reached. Because times of physical exertion had been identified as a possible anxiety-associated cue, the homework assignment for the following week was centered on physical exertion. The client was instructed to plan in his schedule for the next week at least two periods in which he would be taxed physically. It was not at all difficult for him to identify two upcoming activities that would require some extensive physical exertion on his part. One of those was a practice drill for the voluntary fire department and the second was a new task at work that he was going to have to complete within the next week.

The fire department drills were scheduled on 2 different days during the upcoming week, and, of course, the work situation would be a daily event he would have to face until the task was completed. He felt that both of these tasks would require considerable physical exertion on his part and that the fire department drills were quite stressful for him not only because he was not in the best physical shape but also because his performance in those drills was going to be evaluated by the officers of the volunteer fire department.

While Mr. P was concerned about the amount of job-related work and the difficulty of the new work task (he questioned whether or not he would be able to complete the task within the 1-week time limit), he did not feel that it posed any unusual work-related stress for him. Taking advantage of the many opportunities the upcoming week would provide, the therapist and client decided that on at least three occasions during these times of physical exertion, he would practice both his anxiety-induction procedures and his relaxation and cognitive coping strategies. That is, he was specifically to do three self-directed exposure trials during the next week. Whenever possible, he was also to again focus on whether or not he was able to complete the task in spite of the stress and anxiety he experienced during the situation (i.e., he would engage in some hypothesis testing). He would also monitor the types of cognitions and cognitive coping strategies that seemed to be helpful for him during these homework assignments. Of course at other times during the week he was to continue to practice relaxation skills daily, imagery skills at least twice, and to continue careful self-monitoring throughout the rest of the week.

Session 10

At the beginning of Session 10, Mr. P reported that he had experienced a bit of dysphoria for the past couple of days. This dysphoria seemed to be associated with several life circumstances, not the least of which was the fact that he changed his shift at work from a daytime shift to a "graveyard shift." In addition, during the previous week, his 13-year-old son got into some difficulties at school and had generally become more disruptive than was usually the case. And finally, he and his family attempted to go on a camping trip over the weekend in order to "get away from it all for a while and just relax," but the camping trip turned out to be a disaster, primarily because of poor weather and the children's constant complaining about not being able to do what they wanted to do. In spite of these added stresses and difficulties, the client reported only one nighttime panic attack that lasted approximately 5 minutes.

While reviewing his experiences of the previous week, Mr. P noted that the breathing training seemed to be particularly helpful for him, not only in terms of avoiding panic attacks but also in terms of helping him to relax when he noticed that he was becoming tense and anxious. Mr. P also reported two instances of limited symptom attacks, both of which occurred upon waking, and that were defined by general feelings of uneasiness with marked chest tightness and general tension. In both instances, he used cue-controlled relaxation as well as deep breathing to control those limited symptom attacks. The client reported that each of those limited symptom attacks lasted for no more than 2 minutes and reached at most a level of 4 or 5 on the anxiety scale of 0 to 8. He reported that he attempted to use some of the cognitive coping strategies to manage the limited symptom attacks, but he found those techniques to be less helpful than the relaxation and breathing skills.

In reviewing his homework assignments, Mr. P reported that he made substantial progress since the beginning of treatment, especially with relaxation training. However, he was still experiencing difficulty controlling his palpitations and tachycardia when in an anxious situation. He reported that he practiced anxiety provocation by using chest tightness, and that procedure seemed to have reduced the intense manifestation of chest tightness during anxiety episodes. Thus, he felt that the provocation technique was a helpful procedure; however, he reported that both during anxiety attacks and during his use of relaxation exercises, there remained a prominent feeling of "throbbing of his vessels" and palpitations that were not well attenuated with either the relaxation or breathing skills. That the client's focus of attention had shifted from chest tightness to throbbing vessels, palpitations, and tachycardia during anxiety attacks is not atypical. As is often the case, when one irritating symptom is dealt with or eliminated, another symptom or problem surfaces. It is not the case that one symptom is replacing the symptom that was eliminated, but rather that having reduced or eliminated a prepotent symptom, other less manifest symptoms become more obvious. Thus, as the client moves through the hierarchy, he/she redirects the *in vivo* homework assignments to address new symptomatology or new problem areas. Having gathered this new information, Mr. P's therapist then modified the original hierarchy to include the response propositions "throbbing of vessels" and "tachycardia."

After completing the review of the *Weekly Record* and the client's history for the previous week, the therapist then practiced cue-controlled relaxation with the client. The client's response to cue-controlled relaxation was quite good, and again the therapist encouraged the client to practice this technique once a day. He was also instructed to begin to use cue-controlled relaxation in a more consistent fashion to try to deal with anxiety attacks. Next, the therapist had the client again practice anxiety evocation in the office by using chest tightness coupled with shallow breathing. After several successful trials with this technique, interspersed with cue-controlled relaxation, the client attempted to elicit anxiety by imagining and trying to reproduce what he feels when he experiences "throbbing vessels." This experience resulted in an imagery rating of 6 and an anxiety rating of 4.

The next three imaginal hierarchy items were then completed. Each item required two presentations in order to reach the criteria specified in the protocol. Wherever possible the therapist also suggested that the client include as many of the somatic response propositions as possible while imagining the scenes (i.e., chest tightness, tachycardia, shallow breathing, and throbbing of the vessels). The client was instructed to actually attempt to use chest tightness and shallow breathing during the imagination of the scenes if imagination alone was not successful in elevating his anxiety level.

Finally, in this session, the therapist again reviewed the foundation for cognitive management procedures with a heavy emphasis on logical analysis and thinking errors. The client was able to relate several instances during the previous week when his children got into arguments or displayed other kinds of child-management problems that led to significant increases in his anxiety level. He reported that mealtime seemed to be especially problematic at his home and especially stressful for him. The basis of his stress usually had to do with the children "messing around" at the dinner table and constantly arguing with each other about trivial matters. During these mealtimes, he found himself becoming anxious, tense, and occasionally angry, perhaps even losing his temper with his children. Mr. P often found himself worrying that the anger and stress induced by these mealtime disagreements would set off a panic attack. Thus, the therapist targeted these mealtime situations for the next set of self-directed *in vivo* homework assignments.

The therapist suggested that the patient "prepare himself" for mealtime by using his relaxation and breathing exercises to relax for a few moments before the meal starts. It was suggested that this relaxation period might be a good time for him to practice his imagery skills, and rather than focusing on anxiety-provoking images he might focus on pleasant imagery. During the meal, should he feel himself becoming angry, tense, or anxious, he was again to use his relaxation and breathing skills to cope with the situation.

At the same time, he was to try to engage in a logical analysis of the situation in an overt fashion. That is, he was instructed simply to discuss aloud with his family the logic of his feeling angry and tense and to note any errors in thinking or other faulty logic that he discovered during this exploratory time with his family. Because the client reported that almost every meal involved arguing and stress, his homework was to complete these activities at least three times during the next week. The client wrote the instructions for the homework assignments and set up a tentative schedule for completing the assignments with the therapist.

The therapist requested that as soon as the meal was over the client note on the *Weekly Record* his success with instituting the homework practice. The therapist then reviewed the major activities of the current session and checked to see if there was other information the client wanted to share with the therapist. At this point, the client did report that, although it was not indicated on the *Weekly Record*, he was noticing that he was sleeping much better than before treatment started and that he was feeling more rested on waking in the morning even on the days when he had the limited symptom attacks. At this point in therapy, the client felt that treatment was successful, but that as he became less preoccupied with his own anxieties and fears of panic attacks, he was more aware of other difficulties that exist in his life—namely, the parenting problems that we had discussed earlier in this session and dissatisfaction with his job. The therapist assured the client that his experiences are typical of progress in therapy and that as these new problems come to his attention, they will be dealt with in as efficient a fashion as possible. The next therapy session was scheduled for 2 weeks hence because Mr. P and his family were going to spend the following week on vacation.

Session 11

When Mr. P arrived for Session 11, he was in an obviously relaxed and good mood. He reported that they had spent a very pleasant week camping. The past week, both at work and at home, had been quite comfortable for him. On his *Weekly Record*, he reported only one limited symptom attack and no panic attacks. He stated that he was very pleased with the reduction of anxiety episodes that he had experienced over the past 2 weeks, although he still found himself worrying that the panic and anxiety attacks might come back at any time. He also reported that one of his fears was that after he has a panic attack he becomes dysphoric because he sees the return of panic attacks and/or limited symptom attacks as an indication that therapy is not successful. The therapist took advantage of this opportunity to again review with the client the cyclical nature of panic disorder and the fact that he had progressed very well in only 10 sessions. The therapist agreed that he still had substantial work left to do in regard to eliminating his panic attacks and also in developing plans to deal with other problems existing in his life.

Rather than seeing anxiety episodes as indications of therapy failure, the therapist encouraged the client to think of them as good opportunities to practice both the anxiety management skills and the *in vivo* exposure. The therapist also commented at this point that these panic management and elimination skills, like any other skill, needed to be practiced at least occasionally in order to maintain good facility with the skills. Thus, from the therapist's perspective, the fact that the client occasionally has an anxiety episode or indeed even a panic attack is positive because it gives the client an opportunity to practice the very skills that in the long run will help the client manage his life more effectively.

In reviewing the success with the previous *in vivo* self-directed exposure assignments, Mr. P reported that using the relaxation exercises before going to the dining room for the evening meal seemed to help put him in "a little bit more control of himself" during dinner. In addition, he found that using cue-controlled relaxation during dinner also helped him feel less stress when the children began "messing around" at the dinner table. He was able to discuss with the family his anger and impatience about the confusion and havoc that seemed to reign at the dinner table. He said he was surprised to find that his wife and the kids also agreed that dinner was not the most pleasant time for any of them. This led to a discussion of what kinds of procedures the parents could use in order to help the children learn how to behave more appropriately at the dinner table. Although no consensus was reached, the client reported that during the past week the children's behavior at dinner improved at least 100%.

On the *Weekly Record*, the client noted that in spite of the improvement of the children's behavior, he still found himself worrying that dinner times were going to revert to their former level of havoc. He also noted that his tendency to become anxious and angry seemed to be related to his fatigue level and that at times he felt he might have difficulty discriminating anxiety from simple fatigue. In examining the basis for his impatience and anger at dinner time, he first cited the noise level at the dinner table as a primary cause.

On reflection, he also noted that he had always been a "last-minute person," meaning that he tended not to plan very well for imminent activities and as a result always seemed to be in a hurry to get things done. This lack of planning stood in sharp contrast to the client's somewhat compulsive tendency to complete any task started no matter what the situation demanded. These behavioral tendencies also applied to completing dinner. That is, when the children would "mess around" at the dinner table, it generally meant that dinner would be prolonged and not completed in a very efficient manner. Mr. P saw this lack of efficiency in completing dinner as interfering with his ability to complete other tasks and chores.

This insight provided a good opportunity for the therapist to help the client engage in a logical analysis of the self-imposed time pressures that he was experiencing. The therapist guided the client toward examining possible errors in thinking related to the thought that various chores had to be completed by a particular time. This process involved a good deal of decatastrophizing of the consequences associated with not getting common household chores done by a particular deadline.

The therapist also explored with the client ways to change from a "hurried and always catching up" lifestyle to a more "slowed down and planned" lifestyle. During this discussion the client was able to report that at least in some instances, any time pressures he felt were self-imposed time pressures. As an example of this insight, he reported that he decided to buy a new truck, a situation that he was not looking forward to because he disliked negotiating for the purchase of such a large item and in the past had found that such situations made him very anxious. He was fearful that should he become anxious during negotiations for the purchase of this vehicle he might have a panic attack. As a result, he would look foolish in front of the people with whom he was negotiating and have to let his wife deal with the truck purchase.

The therapist again used his plan of shopping for a new truck as an opportunity to structure an *in vivo* self-directed exposure trial. The client agreed to go to at least two truck dealerships during the next week and shop for a truck. While doing so, he was to engage a salesperson in a discussion of the features and prices associated with various models of trucks and he was to attempt to negotiate the best deal that he could for the purchase of a truck. While initially skeptical that he would have the skills to do what was being asked, he did agree to attempt to complete the assignments. The therapist reminded the client that he was to use both his relaxation skills and his cognitive coping strategies during the negotiation process and that it would be helpful if the client could plan the kinds of questions and issues that he felt were important for the negotiation of the purchase of a new truck. Writing the questions down might be useful. He could then rely on these written questions as helpful guides during the negotiation process.

A second homework assignment was suggested. The client had reported that whenever his family went on weekend camping trips, preparing for the trip was always a stressful time, usually because he did not prepare for the trip until "the last minute." Thus, a planned family camping trip provided another good opportunity for Mr. P to work on his anxiety problems. Because the client's family tries to leave for the campsite immediately when the client returns from work, the situation becomes stressful because the children, his wife, and he himself are not packed and ready to leave. The therapist reviewed the importance of planning endeavors and suggested that should it become a stressful situation it would be a good opportunity for Mr. P to again practice his management skills.

As an additional assignment for the upcoming week the therapist also suggested that Mr. P attempt to monitor his fatigue levels as well as anxiety levels in order to examine the correlation between the two. This assignment was suggested because the client had alluded earlier to the fact that fatigue tends to exacerbate his feelings of tension and anxiety.

Session 12

At Session 12, Mr. P reported that he again had a change in his work shift, a situation that usually is stressful for him for a few days; however, this time he reported that he was not particularly`stressed by the work-shift change. In addition, he reported that he had had no panics during the previous week, but he did have three short episodes of what appeared to be general anxiety. During these anxiety episodes, he found the relaxation and breathing exercises to be quite adequate for eliminating or at least reducing the intensity of the anxiety to manageable levels.

Over the previous week, he had noticed that he felt less hurried and under less time pressure. He still found it difficult to set something aside after he had initiated the activity; and, in fact, he felt that he may even be procrastinating in order to avoid having to set the task aside uncompleted. Such reports from clients with GAD are quite common and in fact in this particular case, the "time pressure" issues may simply reflect the GAD features that were recognized during the diagnostic interviews. Generally, while we feel that panic disorder and GAD are independent disorders, they often appear together and indeed may interact in such a way as to exacerbate one another. Because these time pressure problems are stressful for Mr. P, they fall within the purview of the panic treatment protocol in terms of dealing with anticipatory anxiety as a potential cue for initiation of a panic attack.

In regard to the homework assignments, Mr. P reported that his negotiations for a new truck went quite well, although he only undertook one rather than two appointments at sales agencies. He shared with the therapist a list of questions he had written out before he went to the truck agency, and he reported that he was quite tense when he initiated the interaction; however, when he focused on accomplishing his goals for the assignment and became involved in the negotiation process, his anxiety seemed to dissipate. Although he reported that he was not at all satisfied with the sale price or other conditions associated with the negotiations, he was quite pleased that he was able to actually conduct the negotiations in a fashion that he felt was satisfactory.

As he had predicted, the assignment in regard to preparing for the weekend camping trip was quite stressful for him. He reported that he was upset with his wife, who, in turn, was upset with him because he was the only member of the family who had not prepared by packing his belongings for the weekend. He reported that in spite of the tension and the anxiety, he just kept things "moving along." Unlike his wife, who was concerned that it would be very late when they got to the campsite, he was not anxious about getting to the campsite late in the evening. He noted that during this time, he used both breathing and relaxation exercises as well as engaging in some decatastrophizing, for example, asking himself, "Well, what would be so bad about getting to the camp-site after dark? After all, they had set up campsites in the dark several times previously, and, in fact, it might even be a good experience to do it again." In reflecting on the incident, Mr. P reported that he came to understand that it probably was not anxiety or tension that he was experiencing while getting ready to leave for the trip, but rather anger at his wife, who seemed unwilling to understand why he was not becoming upset about their late departure.

Cue-controlled relaxation and the next three items on the imaginal exposure hierarchy were completed during this session. *In vitro* exposure was again practiced, with a focus on chest tightness coupled with shallow breathing to elicit anxiety feelings. In addition, the therapist discussed with the client the role of the experience of throbbing vessels and tachy-cardia that had been discussed in previous sessions as possible cues for panic or anxiety episodes. The client reported that although he occasion-ally still felt as though he were experiencing tachycardia, he was not becoming upset about it. He appreciated that tachycardia did not neces-sarily indicate that he was going to become tense, anxious, or possibly face a panic attack. In fact, he reported that for the past week or so he had been feeling very mellow and that he has noticed that the usual pressures he has at work have been much less stressful for him than they had been in the past. He did, however, report that he was not particularly pleased with his work situation. The therapist again targeted this report for further exploration during the next therapy session.

The *in vivo* assignments that were scheduled for the upcoming week focused on the GAD-like symptoms that the client raised earlier in the session. These behaviors were targeted not only because the client indicated they were problematic for him but also because the number of stressful events and the frequency of both panic and limited symptom attacks had essentially fallen to a level of zero. It is usually at this point in therapy—that is, when panic and anxiety episodes drop to an extremely low level—that we focus on overlearning. Thus, we ensure that clients have learned the management skills and will continue to engage in *in vivo* exposures of one kind or another, even to the extent of creating anxiety-provoking situations. Consequently, the assignments for this upcoming week included first spending one hour working on a relatively major home repair job that the client had been avoiding because he "didn't want to get the job started and then have to quit in the middle of it." Thus the client was instructed to initiate a project on which he was to work for no more than 1 hour. After 1 hour, he was to stop the project and to move on to other kinds of activities. He was not to return to the project until the following day. The client was to note on his *Weekly Record* whether or not stopping in the middle of the project induced any kind of anxiety or stress. If so, he was to note the characteristics of the anxiety and how he dealt with the stress and anxiety generated by that situation. A second assignment was identical to the first except that it involved a different task, and the amount of time to be spent on the second task was only 20 minutes rather than an hour. The client was to complete both of these tasks during the next week.

The client was also instructed to "be on the lookout" for opportunities to use his management and *in vivo* exposure skills. The therapist explained that the client was to be open to the possibility of stressful or anxious situations that occurred in his life and to purposefully try to place himself in those situations rather than attempt to avoid them. The therapist further explained that at this point in treatment it would be very helpful for him to hold off using anxiety management strategies until well after he had spent some minimal amount of time in the stressful or anxiety-provoking situation. The client was to note on the *Weekly Record* a general description of the stressful or anxiety situations that he discovered during the next week.

In discussing the relationship of fatigue to his feelings of anger and anxiety, he clearly came to recognize that in many situations, especially work-related situations, what he was feeling was anger rather than anxiety. In one way or another, he realized that he had been misinterpreting his feelings. He felt that being aware of the attribution in those situations placed him in a position of examining in a more realistic fashion what it was about the situation that was provoking his anger. This theme was also targeted for exploration at the next therapy session.

Session 13

Because of scheduling difficulties, Session 13 took place just 3 days after Session 12. During that time, Mr. P reported that he had had three short panics with three to four symptoms each time. He reported that he did not use his cue-controlled relaxation during any of these panics because he wanted to see if he could handle them without the relaxation techniques. As a result of his attempts to handle the panic attacks in a different way, he noticed first of all that his thoughts could not only influence the intensity of the symptoms that he felt during a panic attack but in fact could bring on the anxiety symptoms. For example, thinking about any day-to-day unpleasantry—or simply anticipating doing anything associated with anxiety or tension—was sufficient to bring on not only feelings of anxiety but also physical symptoms such as tachycardia, chest tightness, and shallow breathing.

As another example, he indicated that his anticipation of completing another firefighting drill at the firehouse was sufficient to induce substantial feelings of anxiety. He did, in fact, engage in some hypothesis testing. He came to realize that he could continue his work in spite of the anxiety and that if he stayed involved in the work situation, eventually the anxiety would dissipate. He also reported that he came to understand that in spite of the anxiety he was not really "out of control." While engaging in this self-reflection, he also came to realize that perhaps his job was much more physically stressful for him than he wanted to admit. He noticed increased physical pain in his back, which he felt was job related. He wondered realistically how long he would be able to stay on the job. Because job satisfaction was targeted as an area for further exploration in the last session, the therapist took advantage of this opportunity to discuss with the client both the positive and negative aspects of his work situation. The client was engaged in a problem-solving process regarding the various alternatives available in regard to his work situation.

While it was clear to the therapist that it would be impossible to deal with the job dissatisfaction issue as well as with some other life circumstances that had become manifest during the course of treatment, the therapist at least acknowledged the existence of these problems for the client at this time and attempted, in a very time-limited fashion, to help resolve these issues. Some of these problems would require additional therapy, and thus the possibility of either referral at the end of treatment or continued treatment focused on these particular situational problems was noted.

Because of the short period of time between sessions, the client reported that he had been able to initiate only one of the assignments agreed upon at the previous therapy session. He did work on a task at home for about 20 minutes and then stopped, went into the house, sat down, and tried to relax for a while before he started another task. He reported that at first he felt extremely uncomfortable but also felt proud that he had been able to complete the assignment. He indicated that he was somewhat surprised that he was able to deal with the situation with as much ease as he did, and, in fact, did not become anxious, as he had predicted he would.

The remaining imaginal exposure hierarchy items were completed, and a review of cue-controlled relaxation was undertaken. The therapist reminded the client that therapy was drawing to a close and explored other potential problem areas with the client. Two basic issues that still seemed problematic for the client were his work situation, as well as some child-management skill deficits that he felt still created stress in his life. He agreed to monitor these stress situations, keeping in mind that therapy focused on these issues may be required. The therapist then initiated a discussion aimed toward developing a generalization practice list. The therapist emphasized the importance of continued practice and generalization of the skills the client had learned in therapy to other situations in his life.

In this regard, the therapist gave the client the assignment of returning next week with a list of activities and/or situations that the client felt would probably occur after the termination of therapy that would provide him with opportunities to continue practicing his exposure and management skills. The client was immediately able to suggest two or three activities and felt that he could generate a rather extensive list without too much difficulty. The therapist asked him to write down his ideas and to return to the next therapy session with a generalization list completed. In addition, the therapist and client decided that he would again initiate an activity that he had been avoiding and then interrupt that activity before it was completed. In this way, he would come to a deeper appreciation of the dynamics involved in his sense of urgency to complete tasks and to meet time pressures.

Sessions 14 and 15

Sessions 14 and 15 were the last scheduled sessions in the anxiety treatment protocol. The major task of these sessions was to deal with any termination issues that had not already been addressed and to prepare the client to continue using skills learned in therapy. The client was instructed to use his generalization list as a guide toward integrating the skills into his everyday life. These sessions were also a time for the therapist to conduct an evaluation of treatment effectiveness with the client.

In Session 14, the client reported that over the previous week, he had two "small" sleep-time panics, both of which lasted only a few minutes and both of which were defined primarily by tachycardia and shallow breathing. The client felt that both of these attacks probably occurred right around the time that he woke up. He did not recall dreaming before he awoke or any other unusual circumstances, and he felt that these were fairly typical of, albeit less intense than, the kinds of experiences he had been having over the previous 10–12 months. He did report the first thing that he became aware of was one of the physical symptoms—that is, either he noticed that his heart seemed to be racing quickly or he noticed that he had some chest tightness. He reported no daytime panics and no limited-symptom attacks except the aforementioned. He noted that he was using the cognitive coping strategies more effectively in dealing with his general background anxiety. His wife noticed that they were having more fun together and that he was much more pleasant to be around. He also stated that he was more aware of other people's tensions and nervousness and felt that he was a more sensitive person.

In both sessions, the therapist and Mr. P reviewed this rather extensive generalization list, which appears in Table 8-4. The therapist discussed with the client various strategies to ensure that he would continue with his skill practices and progress through the generalization list in an efficient and expedient fashion. The client was reminded that the occurrence of panic and limited symptom attacks and/or anxiety episodes should be thought of as good opportunities to practice and sharpen skills rather than as signs of relapse or failure. In fact, the therapist encouraged the client to purposefully continue to place himself in stressful situations and perhaps even make everyday situations a bit more stressful for himself by trying to elicit anxiety with the *in vitro* procedures that were successful previously.

In Session 15, Mr. P reported that during the previous week he had undertaken a major household chore that he had been avoiding for a long period of time—namely, cleaning out his home freezer. He stated that

TABLE 8-4. Mr. P's Generalization List

Events during which panic management skills are to be practiced—at least two practices per week are recommended, as opportunities develop

1. During times of criticism about job performance
2. When faced with a large chore at home
3. When waiting in line at a grocery store
4. When the kids argue and fight, especially at mealtime
5. When I am trying to relax or concentrate on a task and the 4-year-old pesters me
6. When my back troubles me
7. During anxious feelings at sleep time
8. On the long hot drive home after a weekend of camping
9. When the house is messy and disorganized
10. During stress induced by fire drills and evaluation exercises
11. During personal conflicts with spouse or boss
12. While in the dentist's office
13. When I begin to feel tense and anxious
14. Taking the boys camping by myself

Additional activities:
15. Enroll in a child-management class
16. Look into a program for chronic back pain

---

about halfway through the task, he purposefully stopped and ate his dinner before returning to complete the job. He noted that he felt especially good about leaving such a big mess and not finding it stressful enough to disrupt his dinner. His ability to do so seemed to be a major step. Previously, he would not have been able to sit down and enjoy a meal while some major task was left uncompleted. He reported that in his attempts to look for anxiety or stressful situations in his everyday life, he came to realize that he was no longer worried about having a panic attack. Thus, situations that he avoided or entered into with trepidation before treatment no longer elicited strong emotional responses. For example, while he did not like his job any more than he did previously, he was better able to cope with the job stress, and he noticed that this had increased. In addition, he no longer would become panicky or fearful when experiencing physical responses (e.g., an increase in heart rate). Basically, he was no longer afraid that something terrible would happen to him if he became anxious or if he panicked.

During these last meetings, the patient and therapist reviewed a summary of *Weekly Record* from the whole course of assessment and treatment; this review reinforced the client's perceptions of his progress while in treatment. He did voice a typical concern over the possibility of relapse once treatment ended. The therapist addressed the client's concern directly by pointing out that the client had already demonstrated his ability to use those skills in a wide range of situations—thus, the therapeutic focus on and need to continue with practice from the generalization list. Mr. P's rather extensive generalization list and his demonstrated determination to complete practice assignments suggested a good prognosis.

The therapist reminded the client that panic disorder does tend to be cyclical and that he again may be faced with an occasional panic attack; and, of course, stress and anxiety are common experiences in everyone's life. The issue is how one deals with these panics and stress episodes. The client was encouraged to view these anxiety episodes as opportunities to practice and review the skills learned in therapy. On the other hand, should the frequency or intensity of the panic attacks become unmanageable, the client should not hesitate to contact the clinic because occasionally, especially in times of high, prolonged stress, a booster session may be helpful. In any case, regular follow-up sessions are scheduled for 3, 6, and 12 months after treatment ends. This is reassuring to many clients, especially those who are less confident about their ability to continue to progress when therapy ends.

The therapist briefly reviewed the rationale for treatment as well as the major facets of each of the three primary treatment components. The schedule for completing the generalization practices as well as the posttreatment and follow-up reassessments were finalized. Both the client and the therapist recognized that the client was still struggling with some existential problems (e.g., feeling locked into a job he dislikes, declining within the physical limitations imposed by his chronic back problems, and concerns about his children). Wherever possible, the therapist tried to incorporate aids for use in these problem areas into the generalization list (e.g., enrolling in a local parent training class and pursuing a referral to a chronic pain clinic for his back problems). In this way, some attempt was made to help the client deal with other problems that were not specifically targeted in the panic treatment protocol.

Generally, Mr. P evidenced a very positive response to treatment based on questionnaire and self-monitoring data. Furthermore, these therapeutic gains were maintained at a 6-month follow-up. As is typical with many of our patients, he reported feeling an occasional "rumble" during the 6-month period following treatment. He said that some of these rumblings, which referred to clusters of somatic symptoms, might have been recorded as mild panics in times past on his *Weekly Record*. At the present time, however, these rumblings were not disturbing. In other words, Mr. P was no longer anxious over the occurrence of somatic symptoms and had not experienced a panic in 6 months. This kind of report is typical and seems to reflect our conceptualization presented in Chapter 2 that anxiety about panic attacks and the possibility of panic occurring in the future is at the core of panic disorder. Enabling the patient to develop a sense that alarm reactions, if they occur, are manageable and controllable, may well be the most important development in therapy.

Although Mr. P was doing very well at 6 months, occasionally patients follow our advice and call regarding a particularly bad panic attack that they are afraid signals a relapse. Most usually this occurs during a period of very intense stress. For example, one woman who had done very well in treatment was involved in a serious accident in her pickup truck in which a neighbor's child lacerated her face badly on the broken windshield. The stress involved from this incident and its aftermath seemed sufficient to provoke a series of severe panic attacks later that day. Several days later, she called and returned to the clinic. In her case, several booster sessions and some reassurance seemed sufficient to overcome the effects of the traumatic accident.

The overall response to this treatment seems extremely good, based on reports of percentage success as summarized in Chapter 2. Nevertheless, this treatment is still in a preliminary stage of development and we need far more experience with a greater variety of patients under controlled conditions before we can test the limits of generality of effectiveness.

This research is ongoing in our center and elsewhere. In the meantime, the evidence seems sufficient to allow clinicians to utilize this treatment program, adapting it as they wish to relieve the enormous suffering associated with panic disorder.

Appendices

Appendix A. Mr. P's Weekly Record for the Second Week of Pretreatment

Daily ratings of anxiety that you would rate as 4 or above on the anxiety rating scale: Please list any incidents of anxiety that you experience as 4 or above. In addition, please record the letter "P" (following maximum anxiety rating) for an incident that you would label as "panic," which is defined as *sudden rush of anxiety that reaches its maximum level within 10–15 minutes.*

Absent		Mild			Moderate		Much		Maximum
0	1	2	3	4	5	6	7	8	
None		Slightly			Definitely		High degree		As much as you can imagine

Date	Time of onset	Time ending	Situation (Please describe the situation or thoughts that occurred prior to and/or during the anxiety you are reporting) (Symptoms)	Maximum anxiety (and "P" if applicable)	Anxiety at ending time	(Indicate with "X") Non-anxiety-provoking/ nonstressful	Anxiety-provoking/ stressful	What caused this anxiety episode?	Comments
1/5	7 P.M.	7:30 P.M.	Difficulty trying to convince Fire Co. officers to aid me in a necessary job	4	2		X	Difficulty of getting proper help	
1/5	8:00	10:30	Difficulty in controlling our 4-year-old, who will not quiet down to relax; always wants something or is causing trouble	4–6P	2		X	Inability to control child	Tried to relax without medication but failed; 2 Xanax, one at 9:00 and one at 10:15
1/6	9:00	9:30	4-year-old indifferent at breakfast; disciplined and sent to room where screamed and hollered for ½ hour	4	3		X	Conflict with 4-year-old	Ignored to best of ability

(continued)

Appendix A. (continued)

Date	Time of onset	Time ending	Situation (Please describe the situation or thoughts that occurred prior to and/or during the anxiety you are reporting) (Symptoms)	Maximum anxiety (and "P" if applicable)	Anxiety at ending time	Non-anxiety-provoking/ nonstressful	Anxiety-provoking/ stressful	What caused this anxiety episode?	Comments
						(Indicate with "X")			
1/6	10:45	11:30	Toward the end of running, walking exercise period experienced uneven heart beat and heart stoppage	6P	3			Possibly over-exercise	
1/6	12:00	1:30	Went to church with family; general palpitation and tightness in chest area	5	3	X		Fire Co. duties on my mind	Noticeable relief when job was done later in day
1/7	1:00	1:30	Awoke to moderate panic sensations—possibly dreams as cause but can't remember for sure	4P	2		X	Was overtired and tense before bed	Possible worry and difficulty sleeping; took Xanax at 11:30 and resumed sleep
1/7	7 P.M.		Had discipline problems with kids before; also a visit by neighbor though friendly caused heightened anxiety, gradually tightness in chest and neck also	4			X		

Date	Start	End	Symptoms	Time	Rating			Cause/Circumstance	Notes
1/7	6:30	8:30	Irregular and racing heartbeat after supper and slightly before; slight numbness to hands and feet; mild depression after and tiredness	4P	2	X		Many little things to do today and interaction with family	Took Xanax on schedule which helped minimize panic episode
1/7	6:30	10:00	Slight racing of heart; irritable toward children; distracted easily					Unable to relax after supper	Felt good most of the day—even under some bothersome situations
1/7	8:00	9:30	Mild panic symptoms at monthly meeting of firehouse; managed to keep under control; some pleasant feeling because things went well at meeting	4P	3	X		Had to give report; at times ran into opposition but handled it	
1/7	8:30	8:45	Panic surges as I was trying to go to sleep—fairly severe	4P to 6P	—		X	Overtired	Took extra Xanax to help go to sleep
1/7	5:00	5:02	Mild panic surge and muscle tightness in neck area as I turned my head during a safety meeting	4P	2		X	?	Just treated it as a minor annoyance

Appendix B. *Weekly Record* Instructions and Monitoring Forms

You have been given two types of monitoring froms that we would like you to complete *every day*. These forms are very important for three reasons: (1) to give us a better understanding of your anxiety, (2) to provide us with a measure of your improvement throughout treatment, and (3) to help us with our research so that we can keep our treatments completely up-to-date.

Instructions for *Weekly Record* of Anxiety and Depression

We would like you to complete this form once per day, preferably at the end of the day.

After the date put a rating (using the given 0–8 scale) for the average or background level of anxiety—that is, how anxious you felt in general. Next, put a rating for the highest point that your anxiety reached at any time in the day (e.g., if you went to a job interview or thought you'd lost your wallet). The next two ratings refer to your average or general feelings of depression and pleasantness overall throughout the day. We would next like you to list all medications you took that day, including the dose (in milligrams). Finally, please put a rating to indicate, overall throughout the day, how much you worried that you may experience a panic attack. We realize that this feeling will vary from situation to situation, but we would simply like an indication of your overall fear of having a panic attack that day.

Instructions for Panic Attack Record

We would like you to carry these forms with you at all times and to complete them *as soon as possible* after each panic attack. Each time you experience what you consider to be a panic attack, you should note the date, the time it began, and the duration of the actual attack (excluding any earlier or following anxiety). Place a checkmark on the sheet to indicate who you were with and whether or not the panic attack occurred in what was a stressful situation *for you*. For example, if you find going shopping, driving, or going to a party stressful, then this should be rated as such. Rate whether you expected the panic attack or whether it took you by surprise, and also the maximum anxiety that you experienced during the attack. Finally, check any symptoms that you experienced to a reasonable degree during the panic attack.

Make certain you keep all the forms together and give them to your therapist each time you see him/her. If you have any questions about any of the monitoring, feel free to call the clinic.

Weekly Record of Anxiety and Depression

Name _____ Week ending _____

Each evening before you go to bed please rate your *average* level of anxiety (taking all things into consideration) throughout the day, the *maximum* level of anxiety you experienced that day, your *average* level of depression throughout the day, and your average feeling of pleasantness throughout the day. Use the scale below. Next, please list the dosages and amounts of any medication you took. Finally, please rate, using the scale below, how worried or frightened you were, on average, about the possibility of having a panic attack throughout the day.

Level of anxiety/depression/pleasantfeeling

0 ____ 1 ____ 2 ____ 3 ____ 4 ____ 5 ____ 6 ____ 7 ____ 8

None   Slight   Moderate   A lot   As much as
                                                                       you can imagine

Date	Average anxiety	Maximum anxiety	Average depression	Average pleasantness	Medication type, dose, number (mg)	Fear of panic attack

Panic Attack Record

```
                                    Name _____
Date _____  Time _____  Duration _____ (minutes)
With: Spouse _____  Friend _____  Stranger _____  Alone _____
Stressful situation: Yes/No              Expected: Yes/No
Maximum anxiety (circle)
    0 ____ 1 ____ 2 ____ 3 ____ 4 ____ 5 ____ 6 ____ 7 ____ 8
   None                    Moderate                    Extreme
Sensations (check)
   Pounding heart           ____    Nausea                    ____
   Tight/painful chest      ____    Unreality                 ____
   Breathless               ____    Numb/tingle               ____
   Dizzy                    ____    Hot/cold flash            ____
   Trembling                ____    Fear of dying             ____
   Sweating                 ____    Fear of going crazy       ____
   Choking                  ____    Fear of losing control    ____
```

Appendix C. Mr. P's Daily Relaxation Practice

Name Mr. P   Week of 5/14/ to 5/20/   Date 5/14/

Relaxation rating: Rate the *change* in your level of relaxation or tension after practice session.

-10	-9	-8	-7	-6	-5	-4	-3	-2	-1	0	+1	+2	+3	+4	+5	+6	+7	+8	+9	+10
Extreme increase in tension					Moderate increase in tension					No change					Moderate increase in relaxation					Extreme increase in relaxation

Day	Date	Time	Anxiety (0–8)		Relaxation rating	Experience during practice (thoughts, feelings, etc.)
Tues.	5/14/	Practice 1 10.00 A.M.	Before 3	After 1	+2	1. Went to sleep easily again; didn't complete exercises.
		Practice 2	Before	After		
Wed.	5/15/	Practice 1 9.55 A.M.	Before 3	After 1	+2	1. A little uptight and jittery even during practice.
	"	Practice 2 12:30 P.M.	Before 3	After 1		2. Slight panic during stomach muscle exercise.
Thurs.	5/16/	Practice 1 8.30 A.M.	Before 3	After 1	+2	1. Despite things on mind, went to sleep easily.
	"	Practice 2 12:00 mid	Before 3	After 1	+2	2. Relaxed in chair after exercises till 1:00 A.M.

(continued)

Appendix C. (continued)

Day	Date	Time		Anxiety (0–8)		Relaxation rating	Experience during practice (thoughts, feelings, etc.)
Fri.	5/17/	Practice 1	9.30 P.M.	Before 2	After 0	+2	Despite being overtired, managed to get to sleep without much trouble.
		Practice 2		Before	After		
Sat.	5/18/	Practice 1	5.00 A.M.	Before 4	After 2	+2	1. Used breathing and arm exercises to relieve panic.
"	"	Practice 2	10:00 P.M.	Before 3	After 1	+2	2. Went to sleep before finishing.
Sun.	5/19/	Practice 1	5.30 P.M.	Before 2	After 1	+1	1. Used breathing and arm exerices to relieve panic.
"	"	Practice 2	9:30 P.M.	Before 3	After 1	+2	2. Slight panic while doing stomach muscle tightening.
Mon.	5/20/	Practice 1	8.45 A.M.	Before 2	After 0	+2	1. Went right to sleep.
"	"	Practice 2	10:00 P.M.	Before 4	After 2	+2	2. Completed exercises; went to sleep.

Appendix D. Therapist Record: Imaginal Exposure Practice

Client _____

Therapist _____

Item/ Date	Presentation #	Clarity (0–8)	Max. anxiety (0–8)	Time*	Negative thoughts, images	Coping strategies	Comments

*If anxiety was signaled, indicate (a) duration of anxiety or (b) maximum time (max.)

References

Adler, C. M., Craske, M. G., & Barlow, D. H. (1987). Relaxation-induced panic (RIP): When resting isn't peaceful. *Journal of Integrative Psychiatry, 5,* 94–112..

Agras, W. S., Sylvester, D., & Oliveau, D. (1969). The epidemiology of common fears and phobias. *Comprehensive Psychiatry, 10,* 151–156.

American Psychiatric Association. (1980). *Diagnostic and statistical manual of mental disorders* (3rd ed.). Washington, DC: Author.

American Psychiatric Association. (1987). *Diagnostic and statistical manual of mental disorders* (3rd ed., rev.). Washington, DC: Author.

Anderson, D. J., Noyes, R., Jr., & Crowe, R. R. (1984). A comparison of panic disorder and generalized anxiety disorder. *American Journal of Psychiatry, 141,* 572–575.

Aronson, T. A., & Craig, T. J. (1986). Cocaine precipitation of panic disorder. *American Journal of Psychiatry, 143,* 643–645.

Ballenger, J. C. (1986). Pharmacotherapy of the panic disorders. *Journal of Clinical Psychiatry, 47,* 27–32.

Barlow, D. H. (Ed.). (1981). *Behavioral assessment of adult disorders.* New York: Guilford.

Barlow, D. H. (1986). In defense of panic disorder with agoraphobia and the behavioral treatment of panic: A comment on Kleiner. *Behavior Therapist, 9,* 99–100.

Barlow, D. H. (1988). *Anxiety and its disorders.* New York: Guilford.

Barlow, D. H. (in press). The classification of anxiety disorders. In G. L. Tischler (Ed.), *Diagnosis and classification in psychiatry.* New York: Cambridge.

Barlow, D. H., Blanchard, E. B., Vermilyea, J. A., Vermilyea, B. B. & Di Nardo, P. A. (1986). Generalized anxiety and generalized anxiety disorder: Description and reconceptualization. *American Journal of Psychiatry, 143,* 40–44.

Barlow, D. H., Cohen, A. S., Waddell, M., Vermilyea, J. A., Klosko, J. S., Blanchard, E. B., & Di Nardo, P. A. (1984). Panic and generalized anxiety disorders: Nature and treatment. *Behavior Therapy, 15,* 431–449.

Barlow, D. H., & Craske, M. G. (1986). *Psychological treatments of panic disorder.* Paper presented at the 94th annual convention of the American Psychological Association, Washington, DC.

Barlow, D. H., & Craske, M. G. (1988). The phenomenology of panic. In S. Rachman & J. D. Maser (Eds.), *Panic: Psychological perspectives.* Hillsdale, NJ: Erlbaum.

Barlow, D. H., Hayes, S. C., & Nelson, R. O. (1984). *The scientist-practitioner: Research and accountability in clinical and educational settings.* New York: Pergamon.

Barlow, D. H., Vermilyea, J., Blanchard, E. B., Vermilyea, B. B., Di Nardo, P. A., & Cerny, J. A. (1985). The phenomenon of panic. *Journal of Abnormal Psychology,* *94,* 320–328.

Barlow, D. H., & Waddell, M. T. (1985). Agoraphobia. In D. H. Barlow (Ed.), *Clinical handbook of psychological disorders: A step-by-step treatment manual* (pp. 1–68). New York: Guilford.

Beaumont, G. (1977). A large open multicentre trial of clomipramine (Anafranil) in the management of phobic disorders. *Journal of International Medical Research, 5,* 116–123.

Beck, A. T. (1988). Cognitive approaches to panic disorder: Theory and therapy. In S. Rachman & J. D. Maser (Eds.), *Panic: Psychological perspectives.* Hillsdale, NJ: Erlbaum.

Beck, A. T., & Emery, G. (1979). *Cognitive therapy of anxiety and phobic disorders.* Manual of the Center for Cognitive Therapy, 133 South 36th St., Philadelphia, PA 19104.

Beck, A. T., & Emery, G. (1985). *Anxiety disorders and phobias: A cognitive perspective.* New York: Basic Books.

Beck, G. T., Laude, R., & Bohnert, M. (1974). Ideational components of anxiety neurosis. *Archives of General Psychiatry, 31,* 319–325.

Benshoof, B. G. (1987). *A comparison of anxiety and depressive symptomology in the anxiety and affective disorders.* Unpublished doctoral dissertation, State University of New York at Albany.

Bernstein, D., & Borkovec, T. (1973). *Progressive relaxation training: A manual for the helping professions.* Champaign, IL: Research.

Biran, M. E., Augusto, F., & Wilson, G. T. (1981). In vivo exposure vs. cognitive restructuring in the treatment of scriptophobia. *Behaviour Research and Therapy, 19,* 525–532.

Biran, M. E., & Wilson, G. T. (1981). Treatment of phobic disorders using cognitive and exposure methods: A self-efficacy analysis. *Journal of Consulting and Clinical Psychology, 49,* 886–899.

Bonn, J. A., Harrison, J., & Rees, W. (1971). Lactate-induced anxiety: Therapeutic application. *British Journal of Psychiatry, 119,* 468–470.

Bonn, J. A., Readhead, C. P. A., & Timmons, B. H. (1984). Enhanced adaptive behavioral response in agoraphobic patients pretreated with breathing retraining. *Lancet, 2,* 665–669.

Borkovec, T. D., Grayson, J., & Cooper, K. (1978). Treatment of general tension: Subjective and physiological effects of progressive relaxation. *Journal of Consulting and Clinical Psychology, 46,* 518–528.

Borkovec, T. D., & Sides, J. K. (1979). The contribution of relaxation and expectancy to fear reduction via graded, imaginal exposure to feared stimuli. *Behaviour Research and Therapy, 17,* 529–540.

Boulenger, J. P., Uhde, T. W., Wolff, E. A., & Post, R. M. (1984). Increased sensitivity to caffeine in patients with panic disorders. *Archives of General Psychiatry, 41,* 1067–1071.

Bowen, R. C., Cipywnyk, D., D'Arcy, C., & Keegan, D. (1984). Alcoholism, anxiety disorders, and agoraphobia. *Alcoholism: Clinical and Experimental Research, 8,* 48–50.

Breier, A., Charney, D. S., & Heninger, G. R. (1985). The diagnostic validity of anxiety disorders and their relationship to depressive illness. *American Journal of Psychiatry, 142,* 787–797.

Broadhurst, P. L. (1975). The Maudsley reactive and nonreactive strains of rats: A survey. *Behaviour Genetics, 5,* 299–320.

Brown, F. W., (1942). Heredity in the psychoneuroses (summary). *Proceedings of the Royal Society of Medicine, 35,* 785–790.

Buglass, P., Clarke, J., Henderson, A. S., Kreitman, D. N., & Presley, A. S. (1977). A study of agoraphobic housewives. *Psychological Medicine, 7,* 73–86.

Burns, L. E., & Thorpe, G. L. (1977). Fears and clinical phobias: Epidemiological aspects and national survey of agoraphobics. *Journal of International Medical Research, 5,* 132–139.

Butler, G. (1986). Exposure as a treatment for social phobia: Some instructive difficulties. *Behaviour Research and Therapy, 23,* 651–657.

Cacioppo, J. T., & Petty, R. E. (1981). Social psychological procedures for cognitive response assessment: The thought-listing technique. In T. V. Merluzzi, C. R. Glass, & M. Genest (Eds.), *Cognitive assessment* (pp. 309–342). New York: Guilford.

Cannon, W. B. (1929). *Bodily changes in pain, hunger, fear and rage.* New York: Appleton.

Canter, A., Kondo, C. Y., & Knott, J. R. (1975). A comparison of EMG feedback and progressive muscle relaxation training in anxiety neurosis. *British Journal of Psychiatry, 127,* 470–477.

Carey, G. (1985). Epidemiology and cross-cultural aspects of anxiety disorders: A commentary. In A. H. Tuma & J. D. Maser (Eds.), *Anxiety and the anxiety disorders.* Hillsdale, NJ: Erlbaum.

Carey, G., & Gottesman, I. I. (1981). Twin and family studies of anxiety, phobic, and obsessive disorders. In D. F. Klein & J. G. Rabkin (Eds.), *Anxiety: New research and changing concepts* (pp. 117–134). New York: Raven.

Cerny, J. A., Sanderson, W. C., & Barlow, D. H. (1984, November). *The effects of cognitive and relaxation treatments on panic and generalized anxiety disorders.* Paper presented at the meeting of the Association for Advancement of Behavior Therapy, Philadelphia.

Chambless, D. L., Caputo, G. C., Bright, P., & Gallagher, R. (1984). Assessment of fear in agoraphobics: The Body Sensations Questionnaire and the Agoraphobic Cognitions Questionnaire. *Journal of Consulting and Clinical Psychology, 52,* 1090–1097.

Chambless, D. L., Cherney, J., Caputo, J. C., & Rheinstein, B. J. G. (1987). Anxiety disorders and alcoholism: A study with inpatient alcoholics. *Journal of Anxiety Disorders, 1,* 29–40.

Chambless, D. L., & Mason, J. (1986). Sex, sex role stereotyping, and agoraphobia. *Behaviour Research and Therapy, 24,* 231–235.

Charney, D. S., & Heninger, G. R. (1985). Noradrenergic function and the mechanism of action of antianxiety treatment. *Archives of General Psychiatry, 42,* 458–467.

Charney, D. S., Woods, S. W., Goodman, W. K., & Heninger, G. R. (1985). *Involvement of noradrenergic and serotonergic systems: Neurobiological mechanisms of human anxiety.* Paper presented at the annual meeting of the American College of Neuropsychopharmacology, Maui, HI.

Chouinard, G., Annable, L., Fontaine, R., & Solyom, L. (1982). Alprazolam in the treatment of generalized anxiety and panic disorders: A double-blind placebo-controlled study. *Psychopharmacology, 77,* 229–233.

Clark, D. M. (1986). A cognitive approach to panic. *Behaviour Research and Therapy, 24,* 461–470.

Clark, D. M., Salkovskis, P. M., & Chalkley, A. J. (1985). Respiratory control as a treatment for panic attacks. *Journal of Behavior Therapy and Experimental Psychiatry, 16,* 23–30.

Cloninger, C. R., Martin, R. L., Clayton, P., & Guze, S. B. (1981). A blind follow-up and family study of anxiety neurosis: Preliminary analysis of the St. Louis 500. In D. F. Klein & J. G. Rabkin (Eds.), *Anxiety: New research and changing concepts* (pp. 137–148). New York: Raven.

Cohen, A. S., Barlow, D. H., & Blanchard, E. B. (1985). The psychophysiology of relaxation-associated panic attacks. *Journal of Abnormal Psychology, 94*, 96–101.

Cohen, M. E., Badal, D. W., Kilpatrick, A., Reed, E. W., & White, P. D. (1951). The high familial prevalence of neurocirculatory asthenia (anxiety neurosis, effort syndrome). *American Journal of Human Genetics, 3*, 126–158.

Cohen, M. E., & White, P. D. (1950). Life situations, emotions and neurocirculatory asthenia (anxiety neurosis, neuroasthenia effort syndrome). *Archives of Research in Nervous and Mental Disease Processes, 29*, 832–869.

Cohn, J. B. (1981). Multicenter double-blind efficacy and safety study comparing alprazolam and diazepam. *Journal of Clinical Psychiatry, 42*, 347–351.

Coryell, W., Noyes, R., & Clancy, J. (1982). Excess mortality in panic disorder: A comparison with primary unipolar depression. *Archives of General Psychiatry, 39*, 701–703.

Coryell, W., Noyes, R., & House, J. D. (1986). Mortality among outpatients with anxiety disorders. *American Journal of Psychiatry, 143*, 508–510.

Craske, M. G., Sanderson, W. C., & Barlow, D. H. (1987). The relationships among panic, fear, and avoidance. *Journal of Anxiety Disorders, 1*, 153–160.

Crowe, R. R., Noyes, R., Pauls, D. L., & Slymen, D. J. (1983). A family study of panic disorder. *Archives of General Psychiatry, 40*, 1065–1069.

Crowe, R. R., Pauls, D. L., Kerber, R., & Noyes, R. (1981). Panic disorder and mitral valve prolapse. In D. F. Klein & J. G. Rabkin (Eds.), *Anxiety: New research and changing concepts* (pp. 103–116). New York: Raven.

Crowe, R. R., Pauls, D. L., Slymen, D. J., & Noyes, R. (1980). A family study of anxiety neurosis: Morbidity risk in families of patients with and without mitral valve prolapse. *Archives of General Psychiatry, 37*, 77–79.

Dager, S. R., Comess, K. A., Saal, A. K., & Dunner, D. L. (1986). Mitral valve prolapse in a psychiatric setting: Diagnostic assessment, research and clinical implications. *Integrative Psychiatry, 4*, 211–223.

Darwin, C. R. (1872). *The expression of the emotions in man and animals.* London: John Murray.

Denney, D. (1980). Self-control approaches to the treatment of test anxiety. In I. Sarason (Ed.), *Test anxiety: Theory, research, and application* (pp. 209–243). Hillsdale, NJ: Erlbaum.

Depue, R. A. (Ed.). (1979). *The psychobiology of the depressive disorders: Implications for the effects of stress.* New York: Academic.

Depue, R. A., & Monroe, S. M. (1986). Conceptualization and measurement of human disorder in life stress research: The problem of chronic disturbance. *Psychological Bulletin, 99*, 36–51.

Derogatis, L. R., Lipman, R. S., & Covi, L. (1973). SCL-90: An outpatient psychiatric rating scale; preliminary report. *Psychopharmacology Bulletin, 9*, 13–25.

deSilva, P., & Rachman, S. (1981). Is exposure a necessary condition for fear reduction? *Behaviour Research and Therapy, 19*, 227–231.

Di Nardo, P. A., Barlow, D. H., Cerny, J. A., Vermilyea, B. B., Vermilyea, J. A., Himadi, W. G., & Waddell, M. T. (1985). *Anxiety Disorders Interview Schedule—Revised (ADIS-R).* Phobia and Anxiety Disorders Clinic, State University of New York at Albany.

Dittrich, J., Houts, A., & Lichstein, K. L. (1983). Panic disorder: Assessment and treatment. *Clinical Psychology Review, 3,* 215-225.

Doctor, R. M. (1982). Major results of large-scale pretreatment survey of agoraphobics. In R. L. DuPont (Ed.), *Phobia: A comprehensive summary of modern treatments* (pp. 203-230). New York: Brunner/Mazel.

DuPont, R. L., Jr., & Pecknold, J. C. (1985). *Alprazolam withdrawal in panic disorder patients.* New research abstracts of the 138th annual meeting of the American Psychiatric Association, Washington, DC.

Emmelkamp, P. M. G. (1982). *Phobic and obsessive-compulsive disorders: Theory, research, and practice.* New York: Plenum.

Emmelkamp, P. M. G., Brilman, E., Kuiper, H., & Mersch, P. P. (1986). The treatment of agoraphobia: A comparison of self-instructional training, rational emotive therapy, and exposure in vivo. *Behavior Modification, 10,* 37-53.

Eysenck, H. J. (Ed.). (1967). *The biological basis of personality.* Springfield, IL: Thomas.

Finlay-Jones, R., & Brown, G. W. (1981). Types of stressful life events and the onset of anxiety and depressive disorder. *Psychological Medicine, 11,* 801-815.

Flor, H., Turk, D. C., & Birbaumer, N. (1985). Assessment of stress-related psychophysiological reactions in chronic back pain patients. *Journal of Consulting and Clinical Psychology, 53,* 354-364.

Freedman, R. R., Ianni, P., Ettedgui, E., & Puthezhath, N. (1985). Ambulatory monitoring of panic disorder. *Archives of General Psychiatry, 2,* 244-250.

Fyer, A. J., Liebowitz, M. R., Gorman, J. M., Compeas, R., Levin, A., Davies, S. O., Goetz, D., & Klein, D. F. (1987). Discontinuation of alprazolam treatment in panic patients. *American Journal of Psychiatry, 144,* 303-308.

Garakani, H., Zitrin, C., & Klein, D. (1984). Treatment of panic disorder with imipramine alone. *American Journal of Psychiatry, 141,* 446-448.

Gelder, M. G. (1986). Panic attacks: New approaches to an old problem. *British Journal of Psychiatry, 149,* 346-352.

Gitlan, B., Martin, M., Shear, K., Frances, A., Ball G., & Josephson, S. (1985). Behavior therapy for panic disorder. *Journal of Nervous and Mental Disease, 173,* 742-743.

Gorman, J. M., Fyer, A. F., Gliklich, J., King, D., & Klein, D. F. (1981). Effect of imipramine on prolapsed mitral valves of patients with panic disorder. *American Journal of Psychiatry, 138,* 977-978.

Gray, J. A. (1982). *The neuropsychology of anxiety disorders.* New York: Oxford.

Griez, E., & van den Hout, M. A. (1983). Treatment of phobophobia by exposure to CO_2-induced anxiety symptoms. *Journal of Nervous and Mental Disease, 171,* 506-508.

Griez, E., & van den Hout, M. A. (1986). CO_2 inhalation in the treatment of panic attacks. *Behaviour Research and Therapy, 24,* 145-150.

Grunhaus, L., Gloger, S., & Birmacher, B. (1984). Chlorimipramine for panic attacks in patients with mitral valve prolapse. *Journal of Clinical Psychiatry, 45,* 25-27.

Grunhaus, L., Gloger, S., Rein, A., & Lewis, B. S. (1982). Mitral valve prolapse and panic attacks. *Israel Journal of Medical Sciences, 18,* 221-223.

Hall, R. C. W. (Ed.). (1980). *Anxiety in psychiatric presentation of medical illness: Somatopsychic disorders.* New York: SP Medical & Scientific Books.

Hallam, R. S. (1985). *Anxiety: Psychological perspectives on panic and agoraphobia.* New York: Academic.

Hallstrom, C., Treasaden, G., Edwards, J., & Lader, M. (1981). Diazepam, propanolol and their combination in the management of chronic anxiety. *British Journal of Psychiatry, 139,* 417-421.

Hammen, C., Mayol, A., deMayo, R., & Marks, I. (1986). Initial symptom levels and the life-event-depression relationship. *Journal of Abnormal Psychology, 95,* 114–122.

Harris, E. L., Noyes, R., Crowe, R. R., & Chaudry, D. R. (1983). Family study of agoraphobia. *Archives of General Psychiatry, 40,* 1061–1064.

Harrison, B. J. (1985). *Anxiety provoked ideation in phobic and non-phobic panickers.* Bachelor of Arts (Honors) thesis, University of Winnipeg.

Hartmann, N., Kramer, R., Brown, W. T., & Devereux, R. B. (1982). Panic disorder in patients with mitral valve prolapse. *American Journal of Psychiatry, 139,* 669–670.

Haslam, M. T. (1974). The relationship between the effect of lactate infusion on anxiety states and their amelioration by carbon dioxide inhalation. *British Journal of Psychiatry, 125,* 88–90.

Hauri, P., Friedman, M., Ravaris, R., & Fisher, J. (1985). Sleep in agoraphobia with panic attacks. In M. H. Chafe, D. J. McGinty, & R. Wilder-Jones (Eds.), *Sleep research.* Los Angeles: BIS/BRS.

Heide, F. J., & Borkovec, T. D. (1984). Relaxation-induced anxiety: Mechanisms and theoretical implications. *Behaviour Research and Therapy, 22,* 1–12.

Hillenberg, J., & Collins, J. (1982). A procedural analysis and review of relaxation training research. *Behaviour Research and Therapy, 30,* 251–260.

Hoehn-Saric, R. (1981). Characteristics of chronic anxiety patients. In D. F. Klein & J. G. Rabkin (Eds.), *Anxiety: New research and changing concepts* (pp. 399–409). New York: Raven.

Hoehn-Saric, R., Merchant, A., Keyser, M., & Smith, V. (1981). Effects of clonidine on anxiety disorder. *Archives of General Psychiatry, 38,* 1278–1282.

Holden, A., & Barlow, D. H. (1986). Heart rate and heart rate reliability. *Behavior Therapy, 17,* 26–42.

Hume, W. I. (1973). Physiological measures in twins. In S. Claridge, S. Canter, & W. I. Hume (Eds.), *Personality differences and biological variations: A study of twins* (pp. 87–114). Oxford: Pergamon.

Hutchings, D., Denney, D., Basgall, J., & Houston, B. (1980). Anxiety management and applied relaxation in reducing general anxiety. *Behaviour Research and Therapy, 18,* 181–190.

Izard, C. E. (Ed.). (1977). *Human emotions.* New York: Plenum.

Jacob, R. G., Moller, M. B., Turner, S. M., & Wall, C. L. O., III. (1985). Otoneurological examination in panic disorder and agoraphobia with panic attacks: A pilot study. *American Journal of Psychiatry, 142,* 715–720.

Jacobson, E. (1938). *Progressive relaxation* (rev. ed.). Chicago: University of Chicago Press.

Judd, F. K., Norman, T. R., Marriott, P. F., & Burrows, G. D. (1986). A case of alprazolam-related hepatitis. *American Journal of Psychiatry, 143,* 388–389.

Kahn, R. J., McNair, D. M., Lipman, R. S., Covi, L., Rickels, K., Downing, R., Fisher, S., & Frankenthaler, L. M. (1986). Imipramine and chlordiazepoxide in depressive and anxiety disorders. *Archives of General Psychiatry, 43,* 79–85.

Kane, J., Woerner, M., Zeldis, S., Kramer, R., & Saravay, S. (1981). Panic and phobic disorders in patients with mitral valve prolapse. In D. F. Klein & J. G. Rabkin (Eds.), *Anxiety: New research and changing concepts* (pp. 327–340). New York: Raven.

Kantor, J. S., Zitrin, C. M., & Zeldis, S. M. (1980). Mitral valve prolapse syndrome in agoraphobia patients. *American Journal of Psychiatry, 137,* 467–469.

Kazdin, A. E. (1978). *History of behavior modification.* Baltimore: University Park Press.

Klein, D. F. (1964). Delineation of two drug responsive anxiety syndromes. *Psychopharmacologia, 5,* 397–408.

Klein, D. F. (1980). *Diagnosis and drug treatment of psychiatric disorders.* Baltimore: Williams & Wilkins.

Klein, D. F., & Fink, M. (1962). Psychiatric reaction patterns to imipramine. *American Journal of Psychiatry, 119,* 432–438.

Klein, D. F., & Rabkin, J. G. (Eds.). (1981). *Anxiety: New research and changing concepts.* New York: Raven.

Klein, E., Uhde, T. W., & Post, R. H. (1986). Preliminary evidence for the utility of carbamazepine in alprazolam withdrawal. *American Journal of Psychiatry, 143,* 235–236.

Klosko, J., & Barlow, D. H. (1987). *The treatment of panic in panic disorder and agoraphobia: A clinical replication.* Unpublished manuscript.

Kraft, A. R., & Hooguin, C. A. L. (1984). The hyperventilation syndrome: A pilot study on the effectiveness of treatment. *British Journal of Psychiatry, 145,* 538–542.

Lader, M. H., & Wing, L. (1966). *Physiological measures, sedative drugs, and morbid anxiety.* London: Oxford.

Lang, P. J. (1968). Fear reduction and fear behavior: Problems in treating a construct. In J. M. Schlien (Ed.), *Research in psychotherapy* (Vol. III). Washington, DC: American Psychological Association.

Lang, P. J. (1977). Imagery in therapy: An information processing analysis of fear. *Behavior Therapy, 8,* 862–886.

Lang, P. J. (1985). The cognitive psychophysiology of emotion: Fear and anxiety. In A. H. Tuma & J. D. Maser (Eds.), *Anxiety and the anxiety disorders* (pp. 131–170). Hillsdale, NJ: Erlbaum.

Last, C. G., Barlow, D. H., & O'Brien, G. T. (1984). Cognitive change during behavioral and cognitive-behavioral treatment of agoraphobia. *Behavior Modification, 8,* 181–210.

Last, C. G., & Blanchard, E. B. (1982). Classification of phobics versus fearful nonphobics: Procedural and theoretical issues. *Behavioral Assessment, 4,* 195–210.

Latimer, L. (1977). Carbon dioxide as a reciprocal inhibitor in the treatment of neurosis. *Journal of Behavior Therapy and Experimental Psychiatry, 8,* 83–85.

Leckman, J. F., Weissman, M. M., Merikangas, K. R., Pauls, D. R., & Prusoff, B. A. (1983). Panic disorder and major depression. *Archives of General Psychiatry, 40,* 1055–1060.

Levy, A. (1984). Delirium and seizures due to abrupt alprazolam withdrawal: Case report. *Journal of Clinical Psychiatry, 45,* 38–39.

Lewinsohn, P. M., Hoberman, H. M., & Rosenbaum, M. (in press). A prospective study of risk factors for unipolar depression. *Journal of Abnormal Psychology.*

Ley, R. (1985). Agoraphobia, the panic attack and the hyperventilation syndrome. *Behaviour Research and Therapy, 23,* 79–81.

Liebowitz, M. R. (1985). *Pharmacological treatment of panic attacks.* Paper presented at the annual meeting of the American College of Neuropsychopharmacology, Maui, HI.

Liebowitz, M. R. (1986). *Behavioral approaches to the treatment of agoraphobia and panic: The case for pharmacotherapy.* Invited address presented at the 20th annual meeting of the Association for Advancement of Behavior Therapy, Chicago.

Liebowitz, M. R., Gorman, J. M., Fyer, A. J., Levitt, M., Dillon, D., Levy, P., Appleby, I. L., Anderson, S., Daly, M., Davies, S. O., & Klein, D. F. (1985). Lactate provocation of panic attacks: II. Biochemical and physiological findings. *Archives of General Psychiatry, 42,* 709–719.

Liebowitz, M. R., & Klein, D. F. (1979). Clinical psychiatric conferences: Assessment and treatment of phobic anxiety. *Journal of Clinical Psychology, 40,* 486–492.

Lipman, R. S., Covi, L., Richels, K., McNair, M., Downing, R., Kahn, R. J., Lasseter, V. K., & Faden, V. (1986). Imipramine and chlordiazepoxide in depressive and anxiety disorders: Efficacy in depressed outpatients. *Archives of General Psychiatry, 43,* 68–77.

Lloyd, C. (1980). Life events and depressive disorder review: II. Events as precipitating factors. *Archives of General Psychiatry, 37,* 542–548.

Lum, L. C. (1976). The syndrome of habitual chronic hyperventilation. In O. W. Hill (Ed.), *Modern trends in psychosomatic medicine* (Vol. 3). London: Butterworths.

Mackenzie, T. B., & Popkin, M. K. (1983). Organic anxiety syndrome. *American Journal of Psychiatry, 140,* 342–344.

Margraf, J., Ehlers, A., & Roth, W. T. (1986). Sodium lactate infusions and panic attacks: A review and critique. *Psychosomatic Medicine, 48,* 23–51.

Marks, I. M. (1981). *Cure and care of neuroses: Theory and practice of behavioral psychotherapy.* New York: Wiley.

Marks, I. M., Grey, S., Cohen, S. D., Hill, R., Mawson, D., Ramm, E. M., & Stern, R. S. (1983). Imipramine and brief therapist-aided exposure in agoraphobics having self-exposure homework: A controlled trial. *Archives of General Psychiatry, 40,* 153–162.

Marks, I. M., & Mathews, A. M. (1979). Brief standard self-rating for phobic patients. *Behaviour Research and Therapy, 17,* 263–267.

Marsland, D. W., Wood, M., & Mayo, F. (1976). Content of family practice: A data bank for patient care, curriculum, and research in family practice—526,196 patient problems. *Journal of Family Practice, 3,* 25–68.

Masserman, J. H. (1943). *Behavior and neurosis: An experimental psycho-analytic approach to psychobiologic principles.* Chicago: University of Chicago Press.

Mathews, A. M., Gelder, M. G., & Johnston, D. W. (1981). *Agoraphobia: Nature and treatment.* New York: Guilford.

Mavissakalian, M. (1986). The Fear Questionnaire: A validity study. *Behaviour Research and Therapy, 24,* 83–85.

Mavissakalian, M., Salerni, R., Thompson, M. E., & Michelson, L. (1983). Mitral valve prolapse and agoraphobia. *American Journal of Psychiatry, 140,* 1612–1614.

May, J. R. (1977a). A psychophysiology of self-regulated phobic thoughts. *Behavior Therapy, 8,* 150–159.

May, J. R. (1977b). A psychophysiological study of self and externally regulated phobic thoughts. *Behavior Therapy, 8,* 849–861.

Mazza, D. L., Martin, D., Spacavento, L., Jacobsen, J., & Gibbs, H. (1986). Prevalence of anxiety disorders in patients with mitral valve prolapse. *American Journal of Psychiatry, 143,* 349–352.

McCue, E. C., & McCue, P. A. (1984). Organic and hyperventilatory causes of anxiety-type symptoms. *Behavioural Psychotherapy, 12,* 308–317.

McGuffin, P., & Reich, T. (1984). Psychopathology and genetics. In H. E. Adams & P. B. Sutker (Eds.), *Comprehensive handbook of psychopathology.* New York: Plenum.

McNair, D., & Kahn, R. (1981). Imipramine compared with a benzodiazepine for agoraphobia. In D. F. Klein & J. G. Rabkin (Eds.), *Anxiety: New research and changing concepts* (pp. 69–80). New York: Raven.

McNally, R. J., & Steketee, G. S. (1985). The etiology and maintenance of severe animal phobias. *Behaviour Research and Therapy, 23,* 431–435.

Meichenbaum, D. H. (1975). Self-instructional methods. In F. H. Kanfer & A. P. Goldstein (Eds.), *Helping people change* (pp. 357–392). New York: Pergamon Press.

Michelson, L., Mavissakalian, M., & Marchione, K. (1985). Cognitive and behavioral treatments of agoraphobia: Clinical, behavioral, and psychophysiological outcomes. *Journal of Consulting and Clinical Psychology, 53*, 913–925.

Moran, C., & Andrews, G. (1985). The familial occurrence of agoraphobia. *British Journal of Psychiatry, 146*, 262–267.

Mukerji, V., Beitman, B. D., Alpert, M. A., Hewett, J. E., & Basha, I. M. (1987). Panic attack symptoms in patients with chest pain and angiographically normal coronary arteries. *Journal of Anxiety Disorders, 1*, 41–46.

Mullan, M. J., Gurling, H. M. D., Oppenheim, B. E., & Murray, R. M. (1986). The relationship between alcoholism and neurosis evidence from a twin study. *British Journal of Psychiatry, 148*, 435–441.

Mullaney, J. A., & Trippett, C. J. (1979). Alcohol dependence and phobias: Clinical description of relevance. *British Journal of Psychiatry, 135*, 565–573.

Munjack, D. J. (1984). The onset of driving phobias. *Journal of Behavior Therapy and Experimental Psychiatry, 15*, 305–308.

Munjack, D. J., Rebal, R., Braun, R., Shaner, R., Staples, F., & Leonard, M. (1985). Imipramine vs. propranolol for the treatment of panic attacks: A pilot study. *Comprehensive Psychiatry, 26*, 80–89.

Murray, E. J., & Foote, F. (1979). The origins of fear of snakes. *Behaviour Research and Therapy, 17*, 489–493.

Myers, J. K., Weissman, M. M., Tischler, G. E., Holzer, C. E., Orvaschel, H., Anthony, J. C., Boyd, J. H., Burke, J. D., Jr., Kramer, M., & Stolzman, R. (1984). Six-month prevalence of psychiatric disorders of three communities. *Archives of General Psychiatry, 41*, 959–967.

Nelson, R. O., & Barlow, D. H. (1981). Behavioral assessment: Basic strategies and initial procedures. In D. H. Barlow (Ed.), *Behavioral assessment of adult disorders* (pp. 13–44). New York: Guilford.

Norton, G. R., Dorward, J., & Cox, B. J. (1986). Factors associated with panic attacks in nonclinical subjects. *Behavior Therapy, 17*, 239–252.

Norton, G. R., Harrison, B., Hauch, J., & Rhodes, L. (1985). Characteristics of people with infrequent panic attacks. *Journal of Abnormal Psychology, 94*, 216–221.

Noyes, R., Anderson, D. J., Clancy, J., Crowe, R. R., Slymen, D. J., Ghoneim, M. M., & Hinrichs, J. V. L. (1984). Diazepam and propranolol in panic disorder and agoraphobia. *Archives of General Psychiatry, 41*, 287–292.

Nurnberg, H. G., & Coccaro, E. F. (1982). Response of panic disorder and resistance of depression to imipramine. *American Journal of Psychiatry, 139*, 1060–1062.

Öhman, A., Dimberg, U., & Öst, L. G. (1985). Animal and social phobias: A laboratory model. In P. O. Sjoden & S. Bates (Eds.), *Trends in behavior therapy* (pp. 107–133). New York: Academic.

Orwin, A. (1973). The running treatment: A preliminary communication on a new use for an old therapy (physical activity) in the agoraphobic syndrome. *British Journal of Psychiatry, 122*, 175–179.

Pariser, S. F., Jones, B. A., Pinta, E. R., Young, E. A., & Fontana, M. E. (1979). Panic attacks: Diagnostic evaluations of 17 patients. *American Journal of Psychiatry, 136*, 105–106.

Powell, B. J., Penick, E. C., Othmer, E., Bingham, S. F., & Rice, A. J. (1982). Prevalence of additional psychiatric syndromes among male alcoholics. *Journal of Clinical Psychiatry, 43*, 404–407.

Quitkin, F. M., Rifkin, A., Kaplan, J., & Klein, D. F. (1972). Phobic anxiety syndrome complicated by drug dependence and addiction. *Archives of General Psychiatry, 27*, 159–162.

Rachman, S. (1983). The modification of agoraphobic avoidance behaviour: Some fresh possibilities. *Behaviour Research and Therapy, 21*, 567–574.

Rachman, S. (1984). Agoraphobia: A safety-signal perspective. *Behaviour Research and Therapy, 22*, 59–70.

Rachman, S., Craske, M., Tallman, K., & Solyom, C. (1986). Does escape behavior strengthen agoraphobic avoidance? A replication. *Behavior Therapy, 17*, 366–384.

Rachman, S., & Levitt, K. (1985). Panics and their consequences. *Behaviour Research and Therapy, 23*, 585–600.

Rapee, R. M. (1985). A case of panic disorder treated with breathing retraining. *Journal of Behavior Therapy and Experimental Psychiatry, 16*, 63–65.

Rapee, R. M. (1986). Differential response to hyperventilation in panic disorder and generalized anxiety disorders. *Journal of Abnormal Psychology, 95*, 24–28.

Rapee, R. M. (1987). The psychological treatment of panic attacks: Theoretical conceptualization and review of evidence. *Clinical Psychology Review, 7*, 427–438.

Raskin, M., Bali, L. R., & Peeke, H. V. (1980). Muscle biofeedback and transcendental meditation. *Archives of General Psychiatry, 37*, 93–97.

Raskin, M., Peeke, H. V. S., Dickman, W., & Pinkster, H. (1982). Panic and generalized anxiety disorders: Developmental antecedents and precipitants. *Archives of General Psychiatry, 39*, 687–689.

Razran, G. (1961). The observable unconscious and the inferable conscious in current Soviet psychophysiology: Interoceptive conditioning, semantic conditioning, and the orienting reflex. *Psychological Review, 68*, 81–150.

Rimm, D. C., Janda, L. H., Lancaster, D. W., Nahl, M., & Dittmar, K. (1977). An exploratory investigation of the origin and maintenance of phobias. *Behaviour Research and Therapy, 15*, 231–238.

Rosenbaum, J., Woods, S., Groves, J., & Klerman, G. (1984). Emergence of hostility during alprazolam treatment. *American Journal of Psychiatry, 141*, 792–793.

Roth, M. (1959). The phobic anxiety–depersonalization syndrome. *Proceedings of the Royal Society of Medicine, 52*, 587–596.

Roy-Byrne, P. P., Geraci, M., & Uhde, T. W. (1986). Life events and the onset of panic disorder. *American Journal of Psychiatry, 143*, 1424–1427.

Ryback, R. S., Longabaugh, R., & Fowler, D. R. (1981). *The problem oriented record in psychiatry and mental health.* New York: Grune & Stratton.

Salkovskis, P. M. (1988). Phenomenology assessment and the cognitive model of panic. In S. Rachman & J. D. Maser (Eds.), *Panic: Psychological perspectives.* Hillsdale, NJ: Erlbaum.

Salkovskis, P. M., Jones, D. R. O., & Clark, D. M. (1984). Treatment of panic attacks by respiratory control: Covariation of clinical state and carbon dioxide. *Bulletin of European Physiology and Pathology of Respiration, 20*, 91.

Salkovskis, P. M., Jones, D. R. O., & Clark, D. M. (1986). Respiratory control in the treatment of panic attacks: Replication and extension with concurrent measurement of behaviour and pCO_2. *British Journal of Psychiatry, 148*, 526–532.

Sanderson, W. C., & Barlow, D. H. (1986, November). *A description of the DSM-III—Revised category of panic disorder: Characteristics of 100 patients with different levels of avoidance.* Paper presented at the annual meeting of the Association for Advancement of Behavior Therapy, Chicago.

Sarason, I. G., & Sarason, B. R. (1981). Teaching cognitive and social skills to high school students. *Journal of Consulting and Clinical Psychology*, 908–918.

Seligman, M. (1971). Phobias and preparedness. *Behavior Therapy*, 2, 307–320.

Selye, H. (1976). *The stress of life* (rev. ed.). New York: McGraw-Hill.

Shafar, S. (1976). Aspects of phobic illness: A study of 90 personal cases. *British Journal of Medical Psychology*, 79, 221–236.

Shear, M. K., Devereux, R. B., Kramer-Fox, M. S., Mann, J. J., & Frances, A. (1984). Low prevalence of mitral valve prolapse in patients with panic disorder. *American Journal of Psychiatry*, 141, 302–303.

Sheehan, D. V. (1982). Current perspectives in the treatment of panic and phobic disorders. *Drug Therapy*, 12, 179–193.

Sheehan, D. V. (1985). Monoamine oxidase inhibitors and alprazolam in the treatment of panic disorder and agoraphobia. *Psychiatric Clinics of North America*, 8, 49–62.

Sheehan, D. V., Ballenger, J., & Jacobson, G. (1980). Treatment of endogenous anxiety with phobic, hysterical, and hypochondriacal symptoms. *Archives of General Psychiatry*, 37, 51–59.

Sheehan, D. V., Sheehan, K. E., & Minichiello, W. E. (1981). Age of onset of phobic disorders: A reevaluation. *Comprehensive Psychiatry*, 22, 544–553.

Sheki, M., & Patterson, W. (1984). Treatment of panic attacks with alprazolam and propanolol. *American Journal of Psychiatry*, 141, 900–901.

Slater, E., & Shields, J. (1969). Genetical aspects of anxiety. *British Journal of Psychiatry*, (Spec. Publ. 3), 62–71.

Smail, P., Stockwell, T., Canter, S., & Hodgson, R. (1984). Alcohol dependence and phobic anxiety states: I. A prevalence study. *British Journal of Psychiatry*, 144, 53–57.

Snaith, R. P. (1968). A clinical investigation of phobia. *British Journal of Psychiatry*, 117, 673–697.

Solyom, C., Solyom, L., LaPierre, Y., Pecknold, J., & Morton, L. (1981). Phenelzine and exposure in the treatment of phobias. *Biological Psychiatry*, 16, 239–247.

Solyom, L., Beck, P., Solyom, C., & Hugel, R. (1974). Some etiological factors in phobic neurosis. *Canadian Journal of Psychiatry*, 19, 69–78.

Suinn, R. M. (1977). *Manual: Anxiety management training*. Ft. Collins, CO: Author.

Sweeney, E. R., Gold, M. S., Pottash, A. L. C., & Martin, D. (1983). Plasma levels of tricyclic anti-depressants in panic disorders. *International Journal of Psychiatry in Medicine*, 13, 93–96.

Taylor, C. B., Sheikh, J., Agras, W. S., Roth, W. T., Margraf, J., Ehlers, A., Maddock, R. J., & Gossard, D. (1986). Self report of panic attacks: Agreement with heart rate changes. *American Journal of Psychiatry*, 143, 478–482.

Tearnan, B. H., Telch, M. J., & Keefe, P. (1984). Etiology and onset of agoraphobia: A critical view. *Comprehensive Psychiatry*, 25, 51–62.

Telch, M., Tearnan, B., & Taylor, C. (1983). Antidepressant medication in the treatment of agoraphobia: A critical review. *Behaviour Research and Therapy*, 21, 505–517.

Thyer, B. A., & Curtis, G. C. (1984). The effects of ethanol intoxication on phobic anxiety. *Behaviour Research and Therapy*, 22, 559–610.

Torgerson, S. (1983a). Genetic factors in anxiety disorders. *Archives of General Psychiatry*, 40, 1085–1089.

Torgerson, S. (1983b). Genetics of neurosis: The effects of sampling variation upon twin concordance ratio. *British Journal of Psychiatry*, 142, 126–132.

Tsaung, M. T., & Vandermey, R. (1980). *Genes and the mind. Inheritance of mental illness*. New York: Oxford.

Tyrer, P. J., & Lader, M. H. (1974). Response to propranolol and diazepam in somatic anxiety. *British Medical Journal, 2,* 14–16.

Uhde, T. W., Boulenger, J. P., Roy-Byrne, P. P., Geraci, M. P., Vittone, B. J., & Post, R. M. (1985). Longitudinal course of panic disorder: Clinical and biological considerations. *Progress in Neuro-psychopharmacology and Biological Psychiatry, 9,* 39–51.

Uhde, T. W., Post, R. M., Siever, L. J., Buchsbaum, M. S., Silberman, E. K., Murphy, D. L., & Bunney, W. E., Jr. (1981). Clonidine: Effects on mood, anxiety, and pain. *Psychopharmacology Bulletin, 17,* 125–126.

van den Hout, M. A., van der Molen, G. M., Griez, E., & Lousberg, H. (1987). Specificity of interoceptive fear to panic disorders. *Journal of Psychopathology and Behavioral Assessment, 9,* 99–106.

Van Oot, P. H., Lane, T. W., & Borkovec, T. D. (1984). Sleep disturbances. In H. E. Adams & P. B. Sutker (Eds.), *Comprehensive handbook of psychopathology.* New York: Plenum.

Vermilyea, B. B., Barlow, D. H., & O'Brien, G. T. (1984). The importance of assessing treatment integrity: An example in the anxiety disorders. *Journal of Behavioral Assessment, 6,* 1–11.

Vermilyea, J. A., Boice, R., & Barlow, D. H. (1984). Rachman and Hodgson (1974) a decade later: How do desynchronous response systems relate to the treatment of agoraphobia? *Behaviour Research and Therapy, 22,* 615–621.

Vital-Herne, J., Brenner, R., & Lesser, M. (1985). Another case of alprazolam withdrawal syndrome. *American Journal of Psychiatry, 142,* 1515.

Vittone, B., & Uhde, T. (1985). Differential diagnosis and treatment of panic disorder: A medical perspective. *Australian and New Zealand Journal of Psychiatry, 19,* 330–341.

Waddell, M. T., Barlow, D. H., & O'Brien, G. T. (1984). A preliminary investigation of cognitive and relaxation treatment of panic disorder: Effects on intense anxiety vs. background anxiety. *Behaviour Research and Therapy, 22,* 393–402.

Wade, T. C., Malloy, T. E., & Proctor, S. (1977). Imaginal correlates of self-reported fear and avoidance behavior. *Behaviour Research and Therapy, 15,* 17–22.

Wambolt, M. Z., & Insel, T. R. (1988). Pharmacologic models of anxiety. In C. Last & M. Hersen (Eds.), *Handbook of anxiety disorders.* New York: Pergamon.

Watson, J. P., & Marks, I. M. (1971). Relevant and irrelevant fear in flooding: A crossover study of phobic patients. *Behavior Therapy, 2,* 275–293.

Weiss, K. J., & Rosenberg, D. J. (1985). Prevalence of anxiety disorders among alcoholics. *Journal of Clinical Psychiatry, 46,* 3–5.

Weissman, M. M., & Merikangas, K. R. (1985). *The epidemiology and familial transmission of panic disorder.* Paper presented at the annual meeting of the American College of Neuropsychopharmacology, Maui, HI.

Williams, S. L., & Rappoport, J. A. (1983). Cognitive treatment in the natural environment for agoraphobics. *Behavior Therapy, 14,* 299–313.

Wolpe, J. (1958). *Psychotherapy by reciprocal inhibition.* Stanford, CA: Stanford University Press.

Zitrin, C., Klein, D., & Woerner, M. (1978). Behavior therapy, supportive therapy, imipramine and phobia. *Archives of General Psychiatry, 35,* 307–316.

Zitrin, C., Klein, D., & Woerner, M. (1980). Treatment of agoraphobia with group exposure in vivo and imipramine. *Archives of General Psychiatry, 37,* 63–72.

Zitrin, C., Klein, D. F., Woerner, M., & Ross, D. C. (1983). Treatment of phobias: I. Comparison of imipramine hydrochloride and placebo. *Archives of General Psychiatry, 40,* 125–139.

Index